Table Of Contents

Which goals are available? 1

What's the 7-Day Summary? 1

Daily Activity 2

How do I set or change my goals? 3

Viewing Your Goal Progress 3

    Flex 4

    Flex 2 4

What are active minutes? 4

    Do I earn active minutes if I manually log an exercise or activity? 5

    How do I achieve my active minute goal? 5

What are hourly activity goals? 5

    Why do I have an hourly activity goal? 5

    What is my goal? 6

    Where can I monitor my progress? 6

    Am I reminded about my goal? 6

    How do I change my goal? 6

    Is my daily activity goal related to my hourly activity goal? 7

    If I miss my goal, can I make it up by doubling my steps the next hour? 7

    Do all steps count toward my goal? 7

    What is a reminder to move? 7

    Can I turn off reminders to move when I won't be active? 8

    When will I get a reminder to move? 8

    Can I be reminded to move earlier in the hour? 9

    Will I be reminded to move if I'm asleep? 9

How do I track intervals during my workout? 9

    What are intervals? 9

    How do I set each interval length? 9

    How do I start an interval workout? 10

    How do I know when to start and stop moving? 10

    What stats are displayed during my workout? 10

Where can I see a summary of my workout? 10

What should I know about my heart rate data? 11

    How does my Fitbit device detect my heart rate? 11

    What are the heart rate zones? 11

        Peak Zone 11

        Cardio Zone 11

        Fat Burn Zone 12

        Out of Zone 12

        Custom Zone 12

    Resting Heart Rate 12

    How is resting heart rate measured? 13

    What is max heart rate? 13

    What impacts the accuracy of my heart rate reading? 13

    How do I change the heart rate setting on my Fitbit device? 14

    What impacts my heart rate? 15

    What is PurePulse? 15

    What activities don't work with PurePulse? 15

    Are the PurePulse LED's safe? 15

    How do I turn off the LED lights? 16

    Why don't I always see my heart rate? 16

What is my cardio fitness score? 16

    How do I track my cardio fitness? 16

    What is VO2 Max? 16

    How does Fitbit measure my cardio fitness score? 17

    How do I get a more precise estimate of my score? 17

    How does Fitbit calculate my cardio fitness level? 18

    What do the cardio fitness levels represent? 18

    How do I improve my cardio fitness score? 18

    How do I get the best cardio fitness score during runs? 19

    Can I see my cardio fitness score or level on my Fitbit device? 19

    Why don't I have a cardio fitness score or level? 19

    Can I see my cardio fitness history in the Fitbit dashboard? 20

Why don't I see my heart rate on my Fitbit device? 20
How do I measure and adjust stride length for my Fitbit device? 21
    Calculating Your Stride Length 21
    Changing Your Stride Length 22
What should I know about adventures? 22
    What are different adventures? 22
    How do I start an adventure? 23
    How long does it take to finish an adventure? 23
    How do I use the map? 23
    What happens when I reach landmarks? 24
    Can I share landmarks? 24
    Can I get updates about my adventure? 24
    How do I send messages? (Adventure Races Only) 25
    What is my daily destination? (Solo Adventures Only) 25
    How do I use the journal? (Solo Adventures Only) 25
    What happens when I reach treasures? (Solo Adventures Only) 26
    How do I earn badges? (Solo Adventures Only) 26
What should I know about challenges? 26
    What are the types of challenges? 26
    How do I start a challenge? 26
    Who can participate? 27
    Which stats can participants see? 27
    Can I join a challenge that already started? 27
    Can I invite more friends after a challenge has started? 27
    Do I need a Fitbit device to participate in a challenge? 27
    How do I earn trophies? 27
    Can I share my challenge results with friends? 28
    Are there any steps that won't count towards a challenge? 28
    Do GPS activities count towards challenges? 28
    How do I stop getting notified about challenges? 28
    How do I quite a challenge? 28
    What happens if the challenge participants are in different time zones? 29

What should I know about using my Fitbit tracker with the UnitedHealthcare (UHC) Motion program? 29

    I'm having trouble with my tracker 29

    What is the UnitedHealthcare Motion Program? 29

    Which Fitbit trackers can I use? 30

    What should I know about exercise goals? 30

    What's your exercise goal? 30

    Changing Your Exercise Goal 30

    How do I track my goal progress? 31

How do I track my exercise and activities with Fitbit? 31

    Exercise apps and modes on your Fitbit device 31

    Automatic Tracking 34

    Fitbit App 34

        What data does MobileRun track? 34

        How do I start and stop a MobileRun? 35

    Manually log an exercise 37

How do I customize the exercises on my Fitbit device? 38

Food, Weight & Calories 39

    Can I set a weight goal? 39

        How do I set a weight or body fat percentage goal? 40

        How do I change or delete my goal? 40

    What should I know about food scanning? 41

        How do I scan a food item? 41

        Why won't my item scan? 41

        Can I add a barcode to the food database? 42

    How does Fitbit estimate how many calories I've burned? 42

    How do I track my food with Fitbit? 43

        What is a food plan? 43

        How do I start a food plan? 43

        How do I monitor my progress? 44

            Putting together a food plan takes a lot of work. If you feel that you lack the nutrition knowledge to compose a good food plan, it's highly recommended that you speak with your doctor or a nutritionist before starting your new plan. 45

   How do I log food? 45

   Can I scan barcodes to log food? 45

   How do I delete a food entry? 46

   How do I see my macronutrients breakdown? 46

   Do I have to add every ingredient in a meal? 47

   What Type of Food Database Does Fitbit Use? 48

   How do I change the language for my food database? 48

   What is a Calorie Deficit? 48

How do I use Fitbit to track and set goals for my water intake? 48

   Logging Your Water Intake 49

   How do I set a goal for water intake? 49

Sleep 50

What should I know about sleep stages? 50

   What are sleep stages? 50

   How does my Fitbit device automatically detect my sleep stages? 51

   What does each sleep stage mean? 51

   How do I see my sleep stages? 52

   How do I use the sleep stages benchmark? 53

   How can I see the start and end times for my sleep stages? 53

   Can this tell me if I have Apnea or any other sleep disorder? 54

   Why do I see awake minutes? 54

   Why don't I see sleep stages today? 55

   Why don't I see sleep stages for naps? 55

   Can I edit my sleep stages data? 55

   What are some tips for getting a good night's sleep? 55

How do I change my sleep history? 56

   Can I manually log sleep? 56

   Why does my sleep graph say I was asleep when I wasn't? 56

   Why does my sleep graph say I was awake when I wasn't? 56

   How do I edit a sleep log? 56

How do I delete a sleep log? 57

What should I know about setting a sleep schedule? 58

Why should I maintain a consistent sleep schedule? 58

How does Fitbit estimate how much sleep I need? 58

Do I have to set a bedtime and wake-up time target? 58

How are my bedtime and wake-up time targets calculated? 59

How do I meet my bedtime and wake-up time targets? 59

How do I set or change my bedtime or wake-up time target? 59

Do I need to set a bedtime target to receive a bedtime reminder? 60

Health 60

What is female health tracking in the Fitbit app? 60

Why should I use the female health tracking feature in the Fitbit app? 60

What is a menstrual cycle? 60

What are predictions in the female health tracking feature? 61

How does the Fitbit app predict my periods and fertile windows? 61

How accurate are predictions? 61

What are trends in the female health tracking feature? 61

Can female health tracking tell me if I have an unusual cycle or any other disorder? 62

Why do I need to add my birth control method? 62

Can I share my period data? 62

Can I use my female health data for family planning? 63

Can I log ovulation test results in the Fitbit app? 63

Can I log pregnancy test results in the Fitbit app? 63

Is female health tracking available on a child account in a Fitbit family account? 64

How do I use the Fitbit app to track my period? 64

What information can I track in the Fitbit female health feature? 64

How do I set up the female health tracking feature in the Fitbit app? 64

How do I add or remove the female health tracking tile in the Fitbit app? 64

How do I add, edit or delete a period in the Fitbit app? 65

How do I confirm a predicted period in the Fitbit app? 65

How do I log or delete female health details? 66

Can I edit a fertile window in the Fitbit app? 66

How do I read the female health tracking calendar in the Fitbit app? 66

How do I change the day of the week my calendar starts to Monday? 67

What should I know before tracking my period with Fitbit? 67

Why can't I log or edit a period or female health details in the Fitbit app? 68

How can I see trends in my period data? 68

How can I edit my female health settings? 68

Can the Fitbit app remind me when my period will start? 69

Can I edit my average cycle or period length? 69

What do the female health icons mean on the Fitbit app dashboard? 70

Why do my period and fertile windows overlap? 72

How do I log bleeding between my periods? 72

Do I see a period on the Fitbit female health calendar if I log flow details? 72

How do I confirm my period if it arrives early? 72

How can I see my period information on my Fitbit watch? 72

Can I see my cycle information on the Fitbit.com dashboard? 72

How do I add previously tracked cycle information to the Fitbit app? 72

Fitbit Pay 72

What is Fitbit Pay? 73

What banks support Fitbit Pay? 73

How does Fitbit Pay work? 75

Which Fitbit devices work with Fitbit Pay? 76

Anything else you should know? 76

Which goals are available?

Fitbit app offers many health and fitness goals that can help you live a healthy and active life. The following are the goals that the Fitbit app currently offers:

- **Daily Activity**: Start by choosing a goal such as steps taken, active minutes or calories burned. You will feel your tracker vibrate when you have achieved your goal.
- **Exercise**: You can set a target for the number of days per week that you would like to work-out and track your progress using your exercise history.
- **Weight**: Fitbit track offers great help to achieve your weight goals! It's possible to set goals for losing, gaining or maintaining weight. You weight can be captured using Fitbit Aria or you can also manually log your daily weigh-ins. You also have the option to add a goal for your body fat percentage.
- **Water**: Consuming enough water can keep you safe from many health problems. You can use your Fitbit app to track your daily water consumption goal.
- **Food**: Sticking to a good food plan is a great way to achieve your fitness goals. You can create a Fitbit food plan to track your daily calorie input and output. It's also possible to set a daily calorie goal instead of a food plan in the Fitbit app for iOS.
- **Sleep**: Getting enough sleep is an integral part of a healthy lifestyle. You can choose how many hours per night you wish to sleep and monitor your progress in your sleep logs.

What's the 7-Day Summary?

Android and Windows 10 users have the ability to track and view their progress over the past week using the 7-Day Summary in the Fitbit app. There's no need to set goals to receive a 7-Day Summary.

You can smartly use your 7-Day Summary to make adjustments to your goals. Carefully review your summary and maintain your goals based on whether you met or even surpassed your objectives.

You can find your 7-Day Summary by tapping or clicking the Account icon ( ) from the dashboard of your Fitbit app.

Note that the 7-Day Summary is currently not available in the Fitbit app for iOS.

Daily Activity

You can set a daily goal and watch your progress throughout the day. When you reach your goal, your Fitbit device will vibrate and then flash in celebration.

The following will help you to understand how different goals are available for each device. However please consider that, daily goals are not available for Fitbit One and Fitbit Zip trackers.

Device	Goal
Fitbit Blaze	Steps
Fitbit Charge	Floors
Fitbit Charge HR	Distance
Fitbit Surge	Calories burned
	Steps
	Floors
Fitbit Charge 2	Distance
Fitbit Ionic	Calories burned
Fitbit Versa	Active minutes
	Steps
Fitbit Alta	Distance
Fitbit Alta HR	Calories burned
Fitbit Flex 2	Active minutes
	Steps
	Distance
Fitbit Flex	Calories burned
	Steps
Fitbit Ace	Active minutes

How do I set or change my goals?

It's important to set realistic goals to make sure that you enjoy living a healthy and active lifestyle. The Fitbit app provides guidance when creating goals through a series of questions.

You will be prompted to set a goal when you first create your account and at other times in your fitness journey. You can download the Fitbit app from one of these locations depending on the type of your device:

- Apple devices: Apple App Store (https://itunes.apple.com/us/app/fitbit-activity-calorie-tracker/id462638897?mt=8&ign-mpt=uo%3D4)
- Android Devices: Google Play Store (https://play.google.com/store/apps/details?id=com.fitbit.FitbitMobile)
- Windows 10 phones, tablets and computers: Microsoft Store (https://www.microsoft.com/en-us/store/p/fitbit/9wzdncrfj1xx)

You still have the option skip guided (personal) goal setting and make a change at any time by following these steps:

1. Start by clicking the Account icon ( ) from the dashboard of your Fitbit app.
2. Then scroll to the **Goals** section.
3. Tap the goal you wish to view or adjust.
4. Finally, tap the individual element of the goal and follow the onscreen instructions to adjust it.

Ensure that you sync your tracker after changing a goal for those changes to take effect. It's also possible to set and manage your goals using the fitbit.com dashboard. However, you can only access personalized guidance through the Fitbit app.

Viewing Your Goal Progress

The progress bar on your Fitbit screen, indicates know how close you are to reaching your goal. Flex and Flex 2 work differently.

Flex
By tapping the tracker twice, you can see the goal progress on an original flex. Each light represents 20% of your goal and a blinking light represents the ongoing segment.
If two light are on and the third light is blinking, it indicates that 40% of your goal is already achieved and you are now reaching 60%

Flex 2
You can see your goal progress on a Flex 2, by tapping your tracker twice with your finger. There one LED indicator light represents 25% of your total goal. And the blinking LED indicator light shows the segment you're currently working on. For an example, if the first two lights are on and the third is blinking, it says that you've reached 50% of your goal and you're on your way towards reaching 75%.

What are active minutes?
There Your Fitbit device recognizes the differences between different activities like; a regular walk, a brisk walk, a cardio workout, a run and etc. And it awards you with active minutes when the activity you're doing is more strenuous.

How do I earn active minutes?
Fitbit devices calculate active minutes using your metabolic equivalents (METs). These METs help to measure the energy expenditure of various activities. METs are widely used as indicators for exercise intensity because it is taking a person's weight into consideration. When your body is at rest, your MET is equal to 1. Your Fitbit device can estimate your MET value in any given minute by calculating the intensity of your activity.

The Center for Disease Control's (CDC's) has a "10 minutes at a time is fine" concept, where the minutes are only awarded to you only after 10 minutes of continuous moderate-to-intense activity. You can view the CDC's recommendations on the CDC website (http://www.cdc.gov/physicalactivity/everyone/guidelines/adults.html).
You can earn active minutes for activities at or above about 3 METs.

There can be instances where the same activity gives you more active minutes one day and fewer active minutes the next day. This happens with the intensity of the exercising. Your active minute total can change due to slight differences of effort taken over the same difference.

Do I earn active minutes if I manually log an exercise or activity?
Fitbit uses a standard MET score and your (optional) calorie burn to calculate active minutes, when you log manually. Your will be awarded with more active minutes for high calorie burn activities. Custom activities are not associated with a MET score, you'll only get active minutes for them if you also log a high calorie burn.

How do I achieve my active minute goal?
According to CDC recommendation of 20-30 minutes of daily moderate-to-intense activity, your default active minute goal is 30 active minutes per day. But you can always change your active minute goal to meet your personal needs.

Note: Fitbit devices that have heart rate sensors are sensitive in recognizing active minutes for non-step-based activities, such as; weight lifting, strenuous yoga, and rowing. When your device can't track your heart rate, in non-step based activities you will get less active minutes.

MET value, burned calories and total active minutes are proportionately related. When you burn more calories, you will get a high MET value, so therefore a higher total active minutes. Green spikes on your calorie graph, after being active for at least 10 minutes, indicate that you're earning active minutes.

What are hourly activity goals?
Cutting back on stationary time is great way to ensure that you're active throughout the day. Hourly activity goals help achieve that.

Why do I have an hourly activity goal?
It is proven by research that prolonged sitting is linked to a significantly higher risk of heart disease, diabetes, obesity, cancer, and depression and also muscle and joint problems. This is further discussed in source (http://www.ll.dlpa.bru.nihr.ac.uk/Sedentary_Behaviour_New_Study-4347.html). Therefore, sitting for long periods of time can still compromise your health even when follow typical exercise guidelines. For more information see here, source

(http://preventdisease.com/news/14/011014_Sitting-Prolonged-Periods-Stalling-Metabolic-Machinery.shtml). You need to move for a few minutes in every hour to reduce the negative effects which are caused by sitting. Further details are in the source (http://www.ncbi.nlm.nih.gov/pubmed/25931456).

You can only detect your stationary time with devices that can automatically detect sleep. This means if you have a Fitbit One or a Fitbit Zip you won't have an hourly activity goal.

What is my goal?
Your hourly active goal is 250 steps per hour. This is equivalent to a few minutes of walking. Your default, goal tracking is from 9:00 am - 6:00 pm, for seven days a week. But you can track your activity by choosing the consecutive hours per day, as required.

Where can I monitor my progress?
You can see the number of hours that you have achieved of your goal on the Hourly Activity tile on your dashboard shows.

You can see whether each hour tracked in the last week was active or stationary by opening the tile to see the graph. When you swipe, you will be able to see your longest stationary period in the second graph. Please note that the time which you are asleep is not included in this graph, and you must be inactive for at least 10 consecutive minutes before that time is considered stationary.

Am I reminded about my goal?
Your Fitbit device will vibrate 10 minutes before the hour ends and show a reminder if you haven't met your hourly activity goal. Reminders aren't available for Fitbit Charge, Fitbit Charge HR, Fitbit Flex, Fitbit One, Fitbit Surge, and Fitbit Zip.

How do I change my goal?
You can't change the number of steps in your Fitbit device. But you can adjust the number of hours per day that you want to meet the goal with reminders in your device. You can choose between five and 14 consecutive hours per day.

Is my daily activity goal related to my hourly activity goal?

Your daily activity goal and your hourly activity goal are independent form each other. For an example your daily goal of 10,000 steps per day, does not either increase or decrease your goal of 250-step per hour.

If I miss my goal, can I make it up by doubling my steps the next hour?

Just like you can't make up for lost time, you can't make up to a missed goal! Each hour has its own goal. Your extra steps will not be counted in for a previous or a future hour.

Do all steps count toward my goal?

Counting is done only for the steps recorded by your Fitbit device. The steps that you manually log on your dashboard or with the use of the MobileTrack feature, aren't being counted towards your hourly activity goal.

What is a reminder to move?

Most wrist-based Fitbit devices are able to remind you when to move. You will be reminded to walk at least 250 steps each hour by these reminders. When you haven't walked 250 steps, you'll feel a vibration and you will see a reminder on your screen at 10 minutes before the hour ends.

You can change the hours and days where you receive a reminder to move. These are the same hours and days your dashboard tracks your 250-step hourly activity goal. This ranges from a minimum of 5 hours to a maximum of 14 hours in a day. For at least one day per week, you can turn off reminders to move if you don't want to receive reminders. Follow these steps to adjust the hours or days you receive a reminder and track hourly activity goals:

FITBIT APP

1. Begin by tapping the Hourly Activity tile on your Fitbit app dashboard, you can see the number of hours that you have to complete 250 steps.

2. By tapping the gear icon ⚙ you can change your reminders to move start and end times or the days you want to receive reminders.

FITBIT.COM DASHBOARD

1. Begin by selecting the gear icon on your fitbit.com dashboard.
2. Then select your device image.
3. By using Reminders to Move, you can adjust the start and end times or the days that you want to receive reminders.

Can I turn off reminders to move when I won't be active?

You can turn off your reminders on your Fitbit dashboard when you don't want to be reminded to move for a certain period of time.

By turning off the notifications on your Charge 2 you can turn off reminders to move. By pressing and holding the button to stop notifications on the clock face you can turn off the reminders to move, then by repeating the same you can turn on reminders to move again. You'll also find a Do Not Disturb menu on your tracker.

Turning reminders to move on or off:

FITBIT APP

1. Begin by tapping the Hourly Activity tile on the Fitbit app dashboard. This is the tile that shows the number of hours you completed 250 steps.
2. You can turn the Reminders to Move on or off by tapping the gear icon
3. Tap the gear icon and turn Reminders to Move on or off.

FITBIT.COM DASHBOARD

1. Begin by selecting the gear icon on your fitbit.com dashboard.
2. Once you select your device image, you can turn reminders to move on or off by selecting under Reminders to Move.

When will I get a reminder to move?

When you haven't moved 250 steps per hour, you'll receive the reminder at 10 minutes to the hour. You can always take extra steps in the next hour but those won't be counted towards your hourly activity goal, neither previous nor future hour.

Can I be reminded to move earlier in the hour?
Unfortunately, you can only receive your reminder at 10 minutes to the end of the hour. This option can't be changed at this time.

Will I be reminded to move if I'm asleep?
You won't receive reminders if your device detects that you're asleep.

How do I track intervals during my workout?
There is a feature in Fitbit Charge 2, Fitbit Ionic, and Fitbit Versa that helps you to complete a series of guided intervals during your workout.

What are intervals?
Intervals are any exercise that alternates between intense bursts of activity followed by periods of lower intensity activity or rest. You can burn more calories by adding intervals to your workouts and it will improve your aerobic capacity. For more information, see source (http://www.mayoclinic.org/healthy-lifestyle/fitness/in-depth/interval-training/art-20044588).

How do I set each interval length?
You can select from 3 ranges of intervals and total number of rounds that you want to complete, before starting your workout:

- Move period: From 10 seconds up to 19 minutes and 59 seconds
- Rest period: From 10 seconds up to 19 minutes and 59 seconds
- Repeat (total number of rounds): 1 to 49 times

Setting your intervals:
FITBIT APP

1. Begin by selecting the Account icon and your device image from the Fitbit app dashboard
2. By selecting Exercise Shortcuts, you can go to Interval Workout and set your intervals. If Interval Workout isn't listed in the menu, you'll need to add it to your exercise shortcuts.

FITBIT.COM DASHBOARD

1. You can set your intervals by logging into your account in your fitbit.com dashboard and selecting the gear icon in the top right corner

2. Then select Settings and then Devices to continue. When you have more than one device, choose Charge 2, Ionic or Versa.
3. By scrolling down to Exercise Shortcuts you will be able to find Interval Workout and here you will be able to set your intervals. If Interval Workout isn't listed, you can add it to your shortcut by selecting Edit Exercise Shortcuts. Then check the box next to Interval Workout and save your changes.

Please consider that when you set the interval lengths and total number of rounds it will remain as the default options until you change them. When you follow the same workout plan often, you won't need to set the intervals for each time.

How do I start an interval workout?
You can start an interval workout, by simply finding the Interval exercise on your Fitbit device.

How do I know when to start and stop moving?
You can know when to start moving when your tracker vibrates and lights up the word "move" on the dimmed screen. You can know when it's time to recover (to stop moving), when your tracker vibrates and lights up the word "rest" on your screen. This pattern will repeat until you complete all rounds.

What stats are displayed during my workout?
During your workout, you will see the following interval stats on your screen:

- Countdown of the time left in your current round
- Number of rounds that remain in your workout
- Total time left in your workout

By tapping your device during the workout you can easily track your other real-time stats including your heart rate and estimated calories burned.

Where can I see a summary of my workout?
Your exercise history gives you a summary of your workout including your total time, max heart ate, and estimated calories burned.

What should I know about my heart rate data?

How does my Fitbit device detect my heart rate?
Your blood volume changes due to the capillary expansions which are caused by a beating heart. In your Fitbit device the PurePulse LED lights have the ability to detect blood volume changes throughout the day. And you can receive your heart rate data automatically and continuously, which are being generated by a finely tuned algorithm. You can know which heart rate zone you are in, by referring to the heart-rate icon that you see on the display. You will notice 3 heart-rate zones in your device.

What are the heart rate zones?
Heart-rate zones are related with different training intensities. Each heart rate zone targets a specific training intensity that can help you to optimize your workout. Your estimated maximum heart rate is used to set the default zones. Your maximum heart rate is being calculated from your Fitbit device, using the formula of subtracting 220 from your age. The following illustrations will give you a thorough idea for these heart zones. Please consider that there can be slight differences between the icons that changes with the device. As an example, one device will show dots where another device will show dashes, instead. For more information about zones, see the American Heart Association's Target Heart Rates article (http://www.heart.org/HEARTORG/GettingHealthy/PhysicalActivity/FitnessBasics/Target-Heart-Rates_UCM_434341_Article.jsp).

Peak Zone
Peak zone, is the high-intensity exercise zone. In peak zone your heart rate is greater than 85% of the maximum heart rate. You can use this zone for short intense sessions that will improve performance and speed.

Cardio Zone
When your heart rate ranges between 70 to 84% of the maximum heart rate, it defines the Cardio zone. This is the exercise zone of medium-to-high intensity. In this zone, you're pushing yourself without straining yourself. This is the target exercise zone for most people.

Fat Burn Zone

In Fat burn zone, your heart rate ranges between 50 to 69% of the maximum heart rate, this is the exercise zone of low-to-medium intensity. And this is a most suitable zone to target if you are new to exercising. This is known as the fat burn zone because you will burn a higher percentage of calories from the fat depositions. However in this zone you will notice a lower the total calorie burn rate.

Out of Zone

As the name suggests when you are out of zone, which means your heart rate is below 50% of the maximum heart rate. Even in this zone, your heart rate will still be elevated but it won't be considered as an exercise.

Custom Zone

When you are targeting a specific heart rate you can customize your own heart rate zone. This is what known as the custom zone. You can begin by tapping the Account icon ( ) From the Fitbit app dashboard and under Heart Rate Zones you can easily enter your custom zone.

On fitbit.com, you can start by logging into your dashboard and tapping the gear icon, which is in the upper right. Then you can enter your custom zone by choosing Settings and then selecting Personal Info.

The heart-rate value will appear in gray on Fitbit Ionic and Fitbit Versa, when your device is looking for a stronger reading.

Resting Heart Rate

Resting heart rate is a proper indication of how healthy your heart is. It measures your heart beats when you are still. According to the American Heart Association website, active people tend to have lower heart rates due to their strong heart muscles. And they don't need to work as hard like less active people. The average resting heart rate is between 60 to 80 beats per minute. And also, your average resting heart rate rises with your age. For more information, see the American Heart Association's All about Heart Rate article (http://www.heart.org/HEARTORG/Conditions/More/MyHeartandStrokeNews/All-About-Heart-Rate-Pulse_UCM_438850_Article.jsp).

How is resting heart rate measured?

Your heart rate when you're awake, calm and comfortable and have not recently exerted yourself is known as the resting heart. Fitbit uses your heart rate data when you're awake and when you're asleep in order to estimate your resting heart rate. Therefore, to achieve the best accuracy, you need to wear your device to sleep.

Usually your resting heart rate is higher than your heart rate while you are asleep. So you shouldn't worry when your resting heart rate shows a higher value than the lowest value that you see in your heart rate graphs.

What is max heart rate?

Max heart rate is used to calculate your different heart-rate zones. Fitbit calculates your max heart rate by subtracting 220 from your age. It is normal for your heart rate to pass the Fitbit-calculated max heart rate during an intense exercising.

When you are targeting a specific heart rate you can create a custom max heart rate instead of using the default. You can begin this by tapping your Account in the Fitbit app dashboard. Then you can customize your max heart rate by selecting an option to change your heart-rate zones.

What impacts the accuracy of my heart rate reading?

Any heart-rate tracking technology, either a chest strap or a wrist-based sensor, its' accuracy is affected by personal physiology, location of wear, and type of movement.

It's better to wear your device from a finger's width below your wrist bone when you're not exercising. To get the most accurate heart rate readings from you Fitbit's PurePulse, you need to wear it on the top of your wrist.

Tips to improve the heart-rate accuracy:

1. You can wear the device higher on your wrist during exercise to achieve more accurate heart-rate readings. There are exercises that cause you to bend your wrist frequently, such as; bike riding or weight lifting. Such exercises can interfere with the heart-rate signal if you wear the watch lower on your wrist.
2. Always wear your Fitbit in a way that it touches your skin.

3. You shouldn't wear your device too tight, because a tight band can restrict the blood flow, and as a consequence your heart-rate signal will be affected. But when you are exercising you need to wear your device slightly tighter than you do in normal times.
4. When you do high-intensity interval training, like; P90X and boxing that causes vigorous and non-rhythmic movements in your wrist, such movements can prevent the sensor from finding your accurate heart rate. Similarly, with exercises such as weight lifting or rowing, your wrist muscles tend to flex in a way that causes the band to tighten and loosen during exercise. In such an incident you can stay still for about 10 seconds to observe an accurate heart-rate reading. Your Fitbit still provide accurate calorie burn readings during these different types of exercise by analyzing your heart rate trends over the course of the workout.

You should turn off heart-rate tracking in your device when you remove it and put it in a pocket or backpack. In such cases the device will give incorrect heart-rate readings because you are moving.

How do I change the heart rate setting on my Fitbit device?
Changing the heart rate setting on all devices except Ionic and Versa:

1. Begin by, tapping the Account icon ( ) from the Fitbit app dashboard
2. Select your device image.
3. You can change the heart rate settings by tapping Heart Rate and then by choosing On or Auto or Off.

(On the fitbit.com dashboard, begin by clicking the gear icon in the top right. Then you can change your Heart Rate settings by selecting option to change under settings)

For most users, the default setting of Auto is appropriate. In this mode your heart-rate tracker will be active when you are wearing the device and it will be inactive when you remove the device. In an instance where your heart rate isn't being tracked even though you are wearing your device, you can choose On as mentioned in the instructions. When you aren't interested in heart rate tracking or when you want to maximize the battery life, you can choose Off from the menu. Begin to change the heart rate settings on Ionic and Versa by opening the Settings app ( ) and then by tapping Heart Rate. For most people the default setting is On. The heart-rate tracker will be active when you are wearing the device and it will be inactive when you remove the device.

What impacts my heart rate?
There are a several factors that affect your heart rate at any given moment. Movement, temperature, humidity, stresses level, physical body position, caffeine intake, usage of medications and different medical conditions are such impacting things on your heart rate. Therefore it is better if you consult your doctor before starting an exercise routine.

What is PurePulse?
You can receive an automatic, continuous, wrist based tracking for all-day health insights and workout intensity with our PurePulse heart-rate tracking technology. It is uniquely designed to measure your heart rate all day, with the use of always-on optical heart-rate sensors. And also our technology can maintain an extended battery life. With PurePulse you get to accurately track workout intensity and calorie burn. And the finely tuned algorithms provide you a clear insight through interactive charts and graphs.

What activities don't work with PurePulse?
PurePulse can't track second to second details of activities with extreme arm motions, such as boxing. However, you can still receive accurate calorie burn readings during these types of exercises via PurePulse because it analyzes your heart-rate trends over the course of the workout.

Are the PurePulse LED's safe?
PurePulse LED lights are on the visible spectrum, similar to the lights in your home or office therefore it is very rare for you to get an allergic reaction to these LEDs. These LED lights have very low power so you won't burn your skin. And these LEDs are programmed to shut down if your device freezes or can't find a signal. You can turn the LEDs off in a PurePulse if epilepsy or any other condition makes you sensitive to flashing lights.

How do I turn off the LED lights?
Begin by finding the Heart Rate setting on your tracker and by turning it off to stop the blinking lights. You can resume your heart-rate tracking by changing the setting to Auto or On.

Why don't I always see my heart rate?
First you need to make sure if you are wearing the device correctly, if you don't see your heart rate on your device. You can try placing the device higher on your wrist during exercise for an improved fit and more accurate heart-rate reading. And also you can try loosening up the device because when you wear it too tightly, your blood flow gets affected, resulting an effect on the heart-rate signal

You will notice your correct heart rate again after a short wait. You can try changing your Heart Rate setting to Auto, which will make your device track your heart-rate when you're moving. This feature is available for all devices except Ionic and Versa. When you select On, which will make your heart rate tracker always active. If you have and Ionic and Versa, you need to make sure that the Heart Rate setting is On.

What is my cardio fitness score?
You can track your overall cardiovascular fitness in the Fitbit app when you have a Fitbit device with heart-rate tracking (except for Fitbit Charge HR and Fitbit Surge).

How do I track my cardio fitness?
Begin by tapping the heart rate tile on your Fitbit dashboard. You will be able to see a heart-rate graph at the top of the screen. By swiping the graph you will be able to the cardio fitness graph. It presents your cardio fitness score (also known as VO2 Max) and cardio fitness level. More information can be obtained by tapping the arrow in the top right.

What is VO2 Max?
VO2 Max gives you an indication of oxygen usage of your body when you're working out at your hardest. This is widely accepted as the gold standard for grading cardiovascular fitness. According to source (https://med.virginia.edu/exercise-physiology-core-laboratory/fitness-

assessment-for-community-members-2/vo2-max-testing/), the higher your VO2 Max, the more fit you are. This metric can also indicate your performance potential for endurance-based activities including running, biking, and swimming. Further details can be found in source (http://circ.ahajournals.org/content/circulationaha/122/2/191.full.pdf).

Your Fitbit device has the capacity to estimate your VO2 Max value for you with less effort and discomfort. Traditionally measuring of VO2 Max is done in a lab where you run on a treadmill or ride a stationary bike until exhaustion. Here a mask is used to determine the VO2 Max which is strapped to your nose and mouth to gauge the amount of air you inhale and exhale. You can see your VO2 Max as the cardio fitness score in your Fitbit device.

How does Fitbit measure my cardio fitness score?

Your cardio fitness score or VO2 Max is determined by your personal information like; resting heart rate, age, sex, weight, and other. You can obtain the best results, when you enter your exact weight in your Fitbit profile. And you can get better resting heart rate estimates when you wear your device to sleep. You will be able to see cardio fitness score as a range unless you use GPS for runs.

How do I get a more precise estimate of my score?

During your runs when you connect your Fitbit device to GPS, it enables the device of detecting the relationship between your pace and heart rate. In this way you can receive a more precise estimation of your score. Individuals with higher VO2 Max have a lower heart rate while running at the same pace compared to individuals with lower VO2 Max.

Therefore it is better if you run at a comfortable pace for at least 10 minutes, while tracking your run with GPS. (You can use Exercise mode or app with connected GPS, if you are using Fitbit Charge 2, Fitbit Blaze and Fitbit Versa. You can use the Exercise app if you are using a Fitbit Ionic). Better results can be achieved when you run on flat terrain as much as possible because your app only consider the flat sections of your run to get your score estimation. You can go on several runs that are at least 10 minutes in length to do a significant change to your score.

How does Fitbit calculate my cardio fitness level?

Your Fitbit uses a combination of your cardio fitness score, your sex and your age to calculate your cardio fitness level. Due to this you will be able to get a holistic approach to track your cardiovascular fitness over time by comparing to other people with similar sex and age range.

What do the cardio fitness levels represent?

You will receive your cardio fitness score out from the 6 cardio fitness levels that range from poor to excellent. As you can see in, source (http://www.ncbi.nlm.nih.gov/pubmed/2405832), these levels are based on the published data and it will help you to get the above mentioned holistic view of your cardio fitness score in same age range and sex as you.

How do I improve my cardio fitness score?

Sometimes your cardio fitness level can go lower than you'd like. This can be caused due to several factors including a stationary lifestyle. According to source (http://www.hopkinsmedicine.org/healthlibrary/conditions/cardiovascular_diseases/risks_of_physical_inactivity_85,p00218/), such a lifestyle brings serious negative effects on long term health like an increased risk for developing high blood pressure and coronary heart disease.

You can improve your score by exercising and by a healthy weight loss. It will only take two to three months to improve your score by up to 20 percent with increased exercising. You can find more information in Kennedy, Phys. of Sport and Exer., 2012. It is recommended by the American Heart Association to practice at least 150 minutes per week of moderate exercise or 75 minutes per week of vigorous exercise or a combination of moderate and vigorous activity in order to improve overall cardiovascular health. Source (http://www.heart.org/HEARTORG/HealthyLiving/PhysicalActivity/FitnessBasics/American-Heart-Association-Recommendations-for-Physical-Activity-in-Adults_UCM_307976_Article.jsp#.V5J97JODFBd) will provide you more details of improving your overall cardiovascular health.

You can achieve a noticeable improvement when you increase moderate exercising with high-intensity intervals. Interval training can be practiced in any workout when you alternate between intense bursts of activity followed by periods of lower intensity activity or rest. Even though both these endurance training and interval training studies demonstrates an increase in your VO2 Max, according to source (http://www.ncbi.nlm.nih.gov/pmc/articles/PMC3774727/), you can achieve more significant improvements from interval training yields. You can start an interval training workout when you have a Charge 2 or Ionic or Versa.

Healthy weight loss is when you lose your weight by lowering your body fat percentage. And unhealthy weight loss is when you lose your weight by lowering your muscle mass. Healthy weight loss contributes to an increase in your cardio fitness score, where an unhealthy weight loss will bring negative effect on your score as explained in source (http://www-hsc.usc.edu/~goran/PDF%20papers/P99.pdf). You can detect a healthy weight loss goal in your Fitbit profile when the graph shows the potential improvement to your score. And you can't detect potential improvement to your score when your weight loss goal would lower your Body Mass Index (BMI) into the underweight range. For more information about BMI ranges, see the American Heart Association (http://www.heart.org/HEARTORG/HealthyLiving/WeightManagement/BodyMassIndex/Frequently-Asked-Questions-FAQs-about-BMI_UCM_307892_Article.jsp#.V648OJMrKL5).

How do I get the best cardio fitness score during runs?
The following tips will help you to get best estimate when you're running with GPS:

- You can go for long runs (at least 10 minutes long) on flat terrain.
- Always try to complete multiple runs that will help you to improve accuracy.
- Since higher-intensity runs provide a more accurate estimate, it's better if you can run at a faster pace. Here you don't have to run at your maximum speed.

Can I see my cardio fitness score or level on my Fitbit device?
Only your Fitbit app will show you the details of your cardio fitness score and level at this time.

Why don't I have a cardio fitness score or level?
You can use these tips when you don't see your level in the Fitbit app:

- Begin by making sure that you've worn your device for at least 1 to 2 days. You can obtain best results with a better resting heart rate estimate, when you wear your device to sleep.
- You can complete multiple GPS runs to have better run-based measurement of your score.

Can I see my cardio fitness history in the Fitbit dashboard?
Unfortunately, your Fitbit dashboard does not store a history of your cardio fitness score at this time.

Why don't I see my heart rate on my Fitbit device?
With the following troubleshooting tips you can change your Fitbit device when it doesn't show your heart rate. After each step try viewing your heart rate to make sure that you have solved the problem.

- Begin by swiping or scrolling to Settings and finding the Heart Rate Tracking in your Fitbit Blaze, Fitbit Surge. You can change the setting to Auto if it's Off.
- Begin by opening the Settings app ( ) and finding Heart Rate in your Fitbit Ionic, Fitbit Versa— You can change the setting to On if it's Off.
- Begin by choosing Auto setting for your heart rate tracking setting in your Fitbit Alta HR, Fitbit Charge 2 and Fitbit Charge HR.

1. FITBIT APP

- Begin by tapping or clicking the Account icon ( )from the Fitbit app dashboard and selecting your device image.
- By tapping or the tracker tile you can make sure that your Heart Rate is set to Auto.
- Then finish by syncing your tracker.

2. FITBIT.COM DASHBOARD

- Begin by logging into your fitbit.com dashboard.
- Set your heart rate to auto by selecting the gear icon in the top right corner, then by selecting Settings and finally by selecting Devices.
- Then finish by syncing your tracker.
- Your tracker needs a solid contact with your arm to track your heart rate reliably so you need to always tighten the band just enough to prevent it from slipping from on your wrist. Your Heart

rate tracking will not work accessory bands of certain kinds, especially if they're loose fitting. You can wear a Fitbit-branded classic or sport band during exercise to achieve optimal results.
- You can move the band to a slightly different position on your arm—a little higher or a little lower.
- You can try changing the setting to On when you still don't get your heart rate with Auto setting. When it is at On setting you can see the green lights on the back of your tracker flash even when you aren't wearing it. This does not indicate a problem with your tracker.
- Then you can Restart your tracker.
- However, if you still can't see your heart rate, contact Customer Support (https://help.fitbit.com/?cu=1).

How do I measure and adjust stride length for my Fitbit device?

Distance is calculated by Fitbit devices through multiplication of your walking steps by your walking stride length and the multiplication of your running steps by your running stride length.

Your stride length is calculated using your height and sex by default.

Fitbit Blaze, Fitbit Charge 2, Fitbit Ionic or Fitbit Versa evaluate that data to update your running stride length automatically when tracking one or more runs using GPS. Make sure that you run at a comfortable speed for at least ten minutes for best results.

If you feel like your distance measurement might be inaccurate, you can follow the steps below to calculate your stride length and add it to your Fitbit account.

Calculating Your Stride Length
Follow these steps to measure your walking stride length:

1. First of all, you must go to a place where you can measure distance accurately. A track or a field will be ideal.
2. Then start walking and count your steps for a particular distance. You must at least walk 20 steps.

3. Take the total distance (in feet) and divide it by the number of steps to find your stride length.

You can use the same method to calculate your running stride. Just make sure that you run instead of walking this time!

Changing Your Stride Length
Make sure that you carefully follow these steps to change your stride length:

- **FITBIT APP**

    1. Begin by tapping or clicking the Account icon ( ) from the dashboard of your Fitbit app.
    2. Then tap or click **Advanced Settings**.
    3. Tap or click **Stride Length**.
    4. Finally, adjust your stride length.

- **FITBIT.COM DASHBOARD**

    1. You must first log into your fitbit.com dashboard and click the gear icon.
    2. Then choose **Settings** followed by **Personal Info**.
    3. Find **Stride Length** under **Advanced Settings**.
    4. You can adjust your stride length by clicking **Set on Your Own**.
    5. Finally, click **Submit** and then sync your device.

What should I know about adventures?

You can stay motivated with the two adventure modes that you have in your Fitbit app: solo adventures (where you can do non-competitive journeys across scenic landscapes) and adventure races (where you are challenged to take competitive virtual races against your friends across real life locations).

What are different adventures?
Your Fitbit currently presents you with two different series of adventures. One is Yosemite National Park and the other is TCS New York City Marathon. Yosemite National Park consists of three trials. And those are the Vernal Falls trail, Valley Loop trail and Pohono Trail, in that order. The New York City Marathon consists of 3 courses. Those are the 3.1-mile

course, the 10-mile and the 26.2-mile course, in that order.

When you are a solo adventure, you can complete the first trail or course (the shortest distance) and unlock the other two trails, which you can complete in any order.

When you are an adventure racer, you won't get the shortest trails. You can only complete the longer trails in any order.

How do I start an adventure?
Begin your adventure by tapping the Challenges tab, from your Fitbit app. You can do a solo adventure by choosing an adventure and then by tapping Start Tomorrow. You can do adventure races, by choosing an adventure and then by tapping Invite Friends in order to invite your Fitbit friends to the race. In an adventure race you can start your adventure, even when the other participants have not accepted your invitation. You can see that the countdown to your adventure which begins at 12:01AM the following day.

How long does it take to finish an adventure?
The duration of both of these adventures, is determined by the number of steps that you have logged each day.

You can complete your solo adventures at your own pace because those aren't time – based. But you will notice that your adventure expires when don't log any activity in 30 consecutive days.

However your adventure races only last a few days depending on the number of steps that you and your friends take. When one of your friends or you crosses the finish line first, it will take 24 hours from that time, for your adventure race to end. You can make sure that all your steps are counted towards the race by syncing your Fitbit device.

How do I use the map?
You can always get a enhanced view of the trail and surrounding of your adventure area zooming in and zooming out on the map. This is available for both types of adventures.

And also you can have a movie like experience by turning your map into 3D, in your Fitbit app for iOS. You can begin by, opening your adventure in the Fitbit app and by tapping the three dots at the top. Then you can continue by turning on the Toggle 3D Map. By tilting the map by sliding with your two fingers up the screen, you can have an advanced view of your adventure route and surroundings. But you might lose your battery power and mobile data quickly with the 3D map.

What happens when I reach landmarks?
You can think of landmarks as milestones along a trail. When you come to a landmark, first tap the icon and then move your phone to left and right to view the panoramic view on your screen.

You're able to view details such as the step count up to that landmark. Solo adventurers also have the option to view the number of calories burned during the journey, up to that point.

Can I share landmarks?
Reaching a landmark in a journey is an accomplishment! There's nothing wrong with sharing it with your friends and followers on social media. Follow these steps to share a landmark:

1. Begin by opening the adventure in the Fitbit app and tapping the landmark you wish to share.
2. Then tap **Share**.
3. You have the option to write a message. Tap **Next** when you're ready.
4. You have the option to share the post to a specific Fitbit community by selecting or to share with all of your Fitbit friends.
5. When it comes to sharing a landmark on social media, simply tap **Share elsewhere** and select the desired social media network.

Some landmarks can be special to you. If you're using an Android or Windows 10 mobile phone, you can also save a landmark photo as your background image or wallpaper.

Can I get updates about my adventure?
You can stay on track on your adventures by opting for push notifications on your phone. If you're having trouble with receiving notifications, try these troubleshooting steps:

1. First check if you have authorized your phone to receive Fitbit push notifications.
2. The make sure that **Do Not Disturb** is turned off on your phone.

3. Furthermore, make sure **Do Not Disturb** is turned off for your adventure: You can achieve this by opening the adventure in the Fitbit app and then tapping the three dots at the top to make sure that **Do Not Disturb** is off.
4. Visit www.fitbit.com/user/profile/notifications and make sure that you've selected to receive mobile notifications for **Challenges**. Then click **Save**.
5. In the Fitbit app, you can turn on the All-Day Sync option in order to receive timely updates about your adventures. It's important to remember that this option may reduce battery life on both your Fitbit device and phone. You can turn on All-Day Sync by following these steps:
   - Begin by tapping or clicking the Account icon ( ) from the dashboard of your Fitbit app.
   - Then tap your device.
   - Finally, find the option to turn on **All-Day Sync**.

How do I send messages? (Adventure Races Only)

When you're taking part in adventure races, you have the ability to send messages to other participants or cheer on a message that a friend posted. You can send or cheer a message by opening your adventure race in the Fitbit app and then tapping **Messages**. Then select post your message or tap **Cheer** below another participant's message.

What is my daily destination? (Solo Adventures Only)

When you're on solo adventures, your daily destination marks your step target for each day of the adventure. Each adventure has a set distance, but your daily destination is personalized and calculated based on the average number of steps you've taken for the past week.

How do I use the journal? (Solo Adventures Only)

The journal is a great tool to keep track of your progress on solo adventures. It includes a summary of the landmarks, treasures and daily destinations you reach every day. You can view it by opening your adventure in the Fitbit app and then tapping **Journal** at the top of the screen.

What happens when I reach treasures? (Solo Adventures Only)
Treasures make traveling between landmarks fun! Once you discovering a treasure, you have until midnight to open it and complete the short task to add it to your collection. These tasks include fun activities such as quizzes, exercises and logging your data in the Fitbit app.

How do I earn badges? (Solo Adventures Only)
Collect and share the badges that you win from solo adventures with price. Once you finish a trail, you'll earn a new badge which you can share with friends and family.

Note that badges aren't currently available for adventure races.

What should I know about challenges?
You can use challenges to stay motivated. You can either compete with friends and family or complete your personal, non-competitive journeys.

What are the types of challenges?
There are five kinds of races in your Fitbit app:

- Daily Showdown: You can compete with others to achieve the most number of steps for a day.
- Weekend Warrior: You can compete with others to achieve the most number of steps over the weekend.
- Workweek Hustle: You can compete with others to achieve the most number of steps Monday through Friday.
- Goal Day: You can compete and reach the daily step goal with your friends or family.
- Adventures: You can choose between non-competitive solo journeys or challenge your friends to the finish line across real life locations.

How do I start a challenge?
You can start a challenge with your Fitbit app for iOS, Android, or Windows 10. You can begin by opening the app and tapping the Challenges tab. Then you can continue by selecting a specific challenge. Then you can invite other players by finding the option that will help you to choose among your Fitbit friends and contacts. You can select from your mobile contacts and any of your Facebook friends who are using the Fitbit app but not yet from your Fitbit friends. You can add any

person as one of your Fitbit friend when you invite them to the challenge from these lists. You can do non-competitive, solo adventure journey by skipping the step for adding friends.

Who can participate?
You can invite up to 30 people to join an adventure race. For all other challenges, you can only invite a maximum of 10 people. You can initiate a challenge and invite your Fitbit friends, and those friends can invite their friends for the challenge that you have initiated.

Which stats can participants see?
The participants in your challenge can see each other's profile photo, total steps your challenge, posted messages, their personal stats, and achievements.

Can I join a challenge that already started?
Your friends can accept an invitation for the challenge that you have created within twenty-four hours. And when people join after the beginning of the challenge, their step data for the entire challenge length will be counted towards the challenge.

Can I invite more friends after a challenge has started?
You can invite other Fitbit friends after a challenge has started. You can begin this by opening the challenge and finding the option to invite other people. Then you can finish by selecting the friends that you want to include in the challenge and send them invitations.

Do I need a Fitbit device to participate in a challenge?
You participate in a challenge even when don't have a Fitbit device. You can do so by getting the Fitbit app and by choosing MobileTrack during setup. You can track basic stats like the steps that you have taken and your estimated calorie burn with MobileTrack.

How do I earn trophies?
You can earn trophies by becoming the first to completing your goal in a challenge. When you achieve a personal best in a challenge or when achieve your step goal for each day of the challenge, you get to earn trophies.

Can I share my challenge results with friends?
You can share your trophy or badge with your friends and family, when u see the challenge results once a challenge is finished and all the participants have synced their data.

Are there any steps that won't count towards a challenge?
You can only take valid steps in your challenge with your Fitbit device or MobileTrack. You cannot use your activities that were tracked through any third-party apps or your manually logged activities in your challenge total.

Do GPS activities count towards challenges?
As long as you have your Fitbit device with you, you can track a GPS activity with MobileRun. MobileRun uses your phone and the Fitbit app to count your steps during a challenge. And you can count these steps in your challenge totals.

And you can count steps from both GPS activities and non-GPS activities towards a challenge when you are wearing a Fitbit device that offers GPS.

How do I stop getting notified about challenges?
You can receive a push notifications or email from your Fitbit to keep you informed and updated on the challenge. You can stop receiving these notifications:

1. Begin by clicking the gear icon in the top right after logging in to your fitbit.com dashboard.
2. You can continue by selecting Notifications under Settings.
3. You can stop the notifications by unchecking the notification(s) that you don't want to receive from Challenges.
4. Finish by clicking Save.

How do I quite a challenge?
You can see your finished challenges for two days. You can't see a finished challenge after two days. For now, you can only quit an active challenge.

You can quit an active challenge by choosing the Quit option after selecting the Options of a particular challenge.

What happens if the challenge participants are in different time zones?

When you are starting a challenge, it begins and ends in your time zone. The participants that are not in your time zone will receive different challenge leaderboard stats than you.

What should I know about using my Fitbit tracker with the UnitedHealthcare (UHC) Motion program?

Fitbit has made tracking daily progress more meaningful by integrating with UnitedHealthcare Motion program's activity goals.

I'm having trouble with my tracker

If you're having trouble setting up the tracker when using the UnitedHealthcare Motion program, you should contact UnitedHealthcare directly through their support website below: https://www.unitedhealthcaremotion.com/Home/ContactUs.

UnitedHealthcare provides assistance with the following problems:

- Signing up
- Logging in
- Linking your Fitbit tracker to your UnitedHealthcare account
- Syncing your steps to your UnitedHealthcare account

What is the UnitedHealthcare Motion Program?

If you're wondering what UnitedHealthcare's Motion Program is, you will find this section very useful. UnitedHealthcare Motion Program is a set of activity goals called F.I.T., which stands for frequency, intensity and tenacity.

If you are using a Charge 2, you can earn up to $4 per day in credits by achieving one or more of the following F.I.T. goals:

- Frequency: You must space out the times that you're active to achieve this F.I.T. goal. You must complete 300 steps within five minutes, six times a day. However, these 300-step sessions must be at least an hour apart.
- Intensity: This goal is a challenge. You must complete 3,000 steps within 30 minutes, at least once per day.
- Tenacity: This goal is to complete at least 10,000 steps per day.

Which Fitbit trackers can I use?
Currently, Charge 2 is the only tracker that's able to sync with the UnitedHealthcare Motion.

What should I know about exercise goals?

Exercise goals are a great way to track your weekly workout routine and stay motivated.

What's your exercise goal?

According to the American Heart Association, it's recommended that you spend at least 30 minutes on moderate-intensity aerobic activity at least 5 days per week.

Your Fitbit exercise goal helps you track the number of days per week you want to exercise. You goal is 5 days per week by default. Any exercise captured in your exercise history will count towards your exercise goal.

Changing Your Exercise Goal
Your exercise goal is set to five days by default. You can change your goal to a different number of days to suit your own targets and to make tracking easy. However you must have a minimum goal of one day.
You have the freedom to change your goal for current and future weeks. However, you aren't able adjust it for past weeks. Follow the steps below to change your exercise goal.
Note that that you can only modify exercise goals using the Fitbit app. Currently, you can't set or change exercise goals using the fitbit.com dashboard.

- FITBIT APPS FOR IOS AND ANDROID
  1. Begin by opening your exercise history by tapping the Exercise tile on the Fitbit app dashboard. It's the tile that says "Track exercise" if you already haven't worked out today. If you've already worked out today, the exercise category will appear on the tile instead (for example, Run or Hike).
  2. Then tap the gear icon in the top right corner and tap your weekly exercise goal to change it.

- FITBIT APPS FOR WINDOWS
    1. Begin by opening your exercise history by tapping the Exercise tile on the Fitbit app dashboard. It's the tile that says "Track exercise" if you already haven't worked out today. If you've already worked out today, the exercise category will appear on the tile instead (for example, Run or Hike).
    2. Then tap the gear icon at the bottom and tap your weekly exercise goal to change it.

How do I track my goal progress?

Begin by tapping the Exercise tile on your Fitbit app dashboard. There's an icon of a man running surrounded by a pentagon shape at the top of your screen. The sides of this pentagon match your exercise goal.

When you exercise on a particular day, another side of the shape fills in. It's also possible to watch over your exercise goals at a glance through your exercise history.

It's a great feeling when you achieve your fitness goals. You will receipt a congratulatory message when you achieve your weekly goal.

How do I track my exercise and activities with Fitbit?

You can track your workouts and other calorie-burning activities with several ways using your Fitbit. This will help you to meet your fitness goals. You can see your daily totals and exercise history by syncing your Fitbit device with the Fitbit app.

Exercise apps and modes on your Fitbit device

Your Fitbit devices have exercise apps and modes that can track specific activities and give you more precise heart-rate data and stats. For example, by selecting spinning activity on your device you will be able to see real-time stats when you are in a spin class. You will get, a workout summary on your wrist depending on your device. And also you can use GPS to track your exercise and keep the route and pace information in your exercise history.

Tracking an exercise on Charge2:

1. Begin by pressing the button until you get to the Exercise screen on your tracker.
2. You can find the exercise of your choice by tapping.
3. Start the exercise by pressing and holding the button. You will see a phone icon at the top, when your phone is connected to both GPS signal and your device. You will see phone icon with a line , when either your tracker is not connected to your phone or your phone is not connected to a GPS signal. You will see a phone icon with an animated dashed line next to it when your phone is trying to find a GPS signal. You need to make sure that the Fitbit app is allowed to run in the background when your phone is running the Android 8 operating system.
4. By tapping your tracker during your workout you can scroll through your real-time stats or check the time of day. You will notice that your maximum heart rate is shown on an indicator next to the number of beats per minute during the exercise.
5. By pressing the button you can pause and resume your workout
6. By pressing and holding the button you can stop recording when you're done with your workout. You'll see a flag icon and a congratulatory message.
7. By pressing the button you can see a summary of your workout results. You will be able to cycle to a different set of stats with each button press. You can view your exercise summary one time.

By syncing your tracker you can store the workout in your exercise history. There you will be able to discover additional stats and data of your route if you used connected GPS.

Tracking an exercise on IONIC & VERSA:

1. Begin by opening the Exercise app (   ) on your watch.
2. You can select the exercise of your choice by swiping.
3. You can select an exercise by tapping it. You'll see the Let's Go! screen. Satellite icon in the top left your device indicates your watch trying to connect to a GPS signal when you chose a GPS exercise. You can use the built-in GPS on Fitbit Ionic and connected GPS on Fitbit Versa. You know that you watch is connected to GPS when your watch says "connected" and the watch vibrates.

4. The watch allows you begin tracking of your exercise by tappin the play icon or pressing the bottom button. You can see 3 real-time stats of your choice on your watch. By swiping from the middle stat you can scroll through your real-time stats. There you can adjust the stats you see in the settings for each exercise. You can see your progress towards your maximum heart rate during the exercise on an indicator next to the number of beats per minute. When your watch is searching for a stronger reading, the heart-rate value appears in gray.
5. By pressing the bottom button you can let your Fitbit know when you're done with your workout or when you want to pause.
6. When you are prompted, confirm that you want to end the workout.
7. By pressing the top button you will be able to see your workout summary.
8. At the end to close the summary screen by tapping Done.

By syncing your watch you can store the workout in your exercise history. There you can discover additional stats and see your route if you used GPS.

Blaze

1. To find the exercise of your choice begin by, swiping to the Exercise screen and tapping it, On your tracker.
2. A gear icon in the lower left corner indicates that the exercise you chose offers connected GPS. You can either turn on or turn off GPS by clicking on the gear icon. You can then return to your exercise by pressing the Back button (left).
3. You'll see the Let's Go! Screen when you tap and select the exercise.
4. A phone icon in the top left is seen when you are choosing a connected-GPS exercise. You will see dots when your phone is looking for the GPS signal. You will know that the GPS is connected when the phone icon turns bright and the tracker vibrates. A weak GPS signal can cause for you to receive inaccurate route and other activity data. When your phone is running the Android 8 operating system, make sure that you allow the Fitbit app to run in the background.

5. Begin to track your exercise by tapping the screen's Play symbol or by pressing the Select button (lower right). You will receive your appears elapsed time with a stopwatch. By tapping or swiping up and down you can scroll through your real-time stats or check the time of day.
6. You can either pause or mark the end of your workout by tapping the pause icon or by pressing the Select button (lower right).
7. By tapping the flag icon or by pressing the Action button (upper right) you will be able to see a summary of your results.
8. You can close the summary screen by tapping Done or by pressing the Back (left) button.

By syncing your watch you can store the workout in your exercise history. There you can discover additional stats and see your route if you used GPS.

Automatic Tracking
With the SmartTrack feature you receive the ability to automatically recognize, identify and select the continuous, high-movement activities which are at least 15 minutes long. This ensures that you get credit for your most active moments of the day. By syncing your device, you can record the basic stats about your activity in your exercise history.

Fitbit App
This feature which is also known as MobileRun works wonders if you Fitbit device doesn't have GPS in case you don't have it with you. With this feature, you are able to map your activity and capture GPS data using the Fitbit app on your mobile phone.

What data does MobileRun track?
Mobile run uses the GPS sensors in your phone to calculate details such as distance, elevation, and your speeds for walking, running or hiking. You are able to access all the data and a GPS map in your exercise history, once the activity is completed and your Fitbit tracker is synced.

If you use MobileRun while wearing your tracker, details such as the steps, active minutes and calories burned that are displayed on your Fitbit dashboard will come from the tracker.

If your trackers is not present, your phone is used to calculate those stats. You are able to view the elapsed distance, time and average pace during the workout. You also have the ability to use the music controls in the Fitbit app.

How do I start and stop a MobileRun?

When it comes to starting and stopping MobileRun, follow the instructions according to the type of Fitbit app you're using.

- FITBIT APP FOR IOS
    1. Begin by tapping the + icon from the dashboard of your Fitbit app.
    2. Then tap **Track Exercise**, followed by taping **Track** at the top of the screen.
    3. From there, you can choose one of the following activities: Run, Walk or Hike.
    4. You can have your phone provide voice cues during an activity. You can enable this feature by tapping **Cues** to set the voice cues you wish to hear and the frequency and volume of the cues.
    5. It's also possible to control the music from the Exercise screen during your activity. You can enable this by tapping **Music Control** and choosing your preferred music settings. You can the ability to skip songs during an activity. However, you're not able to select a specific song.
    6. You can proceed by tapping **Start**. If you would like to view the GPS map during an activity, simply swipe left.
    7. You can finish an activity by tapping the **Pause** button and then tap and holding the **Finish** button. An activity summary will be displayed providing you information about your steps, distance, active minutes and calories burned as calculated using the sensors on your phone.

- FITBIT APP FOR ANDROID
    1. Begin by tapping the + icon from the dashboard of your Fitbit app.
    2. Then tap **Track Exercise**, followed by tapping **Tracking** at the top of the screen.

3. For devices with Android Marshmallow, you must first grant the Fitbit app access to the requested features of your phone.
4. Then choose one of the following activities: Running, Walking or Hiking.
5. You can have your phone provide voice cues during an activity. Enable this by tapping **Use voice cues** and start setting the voice cues you would like to hear as well as the frequency of those cues.
6. You can then proceed by tapping **Start**. If you would like to view the GPS map during an activity, simply swipe left.
7. You can finish an activity by tapping the **Pause** button and then tap and holding the **Finish** button. An activity summary will be displayed providing you information about your steps, distance, active minutes and calories burned as calculated using the sensors on your phone.

- FITBIT APP FOR WINDOWS 10
    1. Begin by tapping the + icon from the dashboard of your Fitbit app.
    2. Then tap **Track Exercise**.
    3. Then choose one of the following activities: Running, Walking or Hiking.
    4. You can have your phone provide voice cues during an activity. Achieve this by tapping **Voice Cues** to set the voice cues you want to hear as well as the frequency and volume of those cues. **Note**: You're not able to have voice cues while music is being played.
    5. You can then proceed by tapping **Start** and tapping **Start** again. If you would like to view the GPS map during an activity, simply swipe left.
    6. You can finish an activity by tapping the **Pause** button and then tap and holding the **Finish** button. An activity summary will be displayed providing you information about your steps, distance, active minutes and calories burned as calculated using the sensors on your phone.

Manually log an exercise

You can manually log an exercise when:

- You forgot to wear your device
- You need to get credits for a calorie-burning activities that aren't measurable by your device or the activities that aren't step-based (i.e. yoga)
- Your tracker doesn't offer SmartTrack or exercise apps or modes
- You want to improve your totals by replacing a recorded activity with manual data

The following section will provide you instructions to manually log an activity.

- **FITBIT.COM DASHBOARD**
1. Begin by logging into your fitbit.com dashboard.
2. You can select Activities by clicking Log at the top of the page.
3. You can either click a common activity or search for one. And also you can Create your own activity by clicking the Create custom activity text that appears below the search field when the activity you need is not in our system.
4. You can enter the duration, distance (if applicable), the start time of your activity and the number of calories burned into your device.
5. By click Log you will be able to see your activity be visible and editable in the Activity History area.
- FITBIT APP FOR IOS
1. Begin by tapping the Exercise tile to open your exercise history on the Fitbit app dashboard. You can recognize this tile which says "Track exercise" or shows how many days you've worked out this week.
2. Then by tapping the stopwatch icon in the top right corner and tapping Log, you can easily tap a recent activity or search for an exercise type.
3. Finish by adjusting the activity details and tapping Add.

You can also log an activity from the home screen when your iOS mobile device supports 3D Touch, by selecting the Quick Action menu accessed by 3D Touch.

- **FITBIT APP FOR ANDROID**
1. Begin by opening your exercise history by tapping the Exercise tile on the Fitbit app dashboard. You can recognize this tile which says "Track exercise" or shows how many days you've worked out this week.
2. Then by tapping the stopwatch icon in the top right corner and tapping Log Previous, you can adjust the activity details
3. Finish by tapping Log It.
- FITBIT APP FOR WINDOWS 10
1. Begin by opening your exercise history by tapping the Exercise tile on the Fitbit app dashboard. You can recognize this tile which says "Track exercise" or shows how many days you've worked out this week.
2. You can select a recent activity or search for an exercise type by tapping or clicking the "+" icon on the bottom.
3. Finish by adjusting the activity details and tapping or clicking Log.

How do I customize the exercises on my Fitbit device?

You can always configure your Fitbit device with an Exercise menu or app to show you only the selected exercises, which interest you from the available exercises. You can choose Workout as your exercise type when a specific exercise isn't available.

Changing or re-ordering the exercises on your Fitbit device:

- **FITBIT APP FOR IOS**
1. Begin by tapping the Account icon ( ) From the Fitbit app dashboard and by selecting your device image.
2. You can add a new shortcut by selecting Tap Exercise Shortcuts and then by selecting an exercise.
3. You can remove a shortcut, by swiping left on an exercise name, then by tapping Delete.
- **FITBIT APP FOR ANDROID**
1. Begin by tapping the Account icon ( ) and selecting your device image from the Fitbit app dashboard.
2. You can select an exercise and add a new shortcut for the selected exercise, from tapping the Exercise Shortcuts and then by clicking the + icon.

3. You can remove a shortcut by swiping left on an exercise name.
- **FITBIT APP FOR WINDOWS 10**
1. Begin by tapping or click the Account icon ( ) and selecting your device image from the Fitbit app dashboard.
2. You can select an exercise and add a new shortcut for the selected exercise, from tapping the Exercise Shortcuts and then by clicking the + icon.
3. You can remove a shortcut by tapping or clicking the trashcan icon.
- **FITBIT.COM DASHBOARD**
1. Begin by logging into your fitbit.com dashboard and clicking the gear icon in the top right corner.
2. When you have multiple trackers on your account, make sure you're focusing on the correct tracker and the select Devices by clicking the Settings.
3. You can choose the exercises you want on your tracker by scrolling down to the Exercise Shortcuts section and then by clicking Edit Exercise Shortcuts.
4. Save your changes by clicking Save. You need to have at least one exercise on your tracker.
5. Finish by clicking and dragging the Row Reorder icons to arrange the exercises in the order you want on your tracker. You will notice your changes in the next time when you sync your tracker.

You can get any existing stats for a removed exercise from your exercise history.

Food, Weight & Calories

Can I set a weight goal?
You can add and track your progress towards a body fat goal as well as goals for losing, gaining or maintaining weight on your Fitbit account.
The food that you consume is a deciding factor of your reaching your weight goals. You can synchronize goals with your Food Plan if you have one.

How do I set a weight or body fat percentage goal?

It's possible that you may be keeping an eye on your weight or body fat percentage or both. Follow these steps to set up a weight or body fat percentage goal:

- **FITBIT APP**
    1. Start by clicking the Account icon ( ) from the dashboard of your Fitbit app.
    2. Then find **Nutrition & Body** under Goals.
    3. Proceed by selecting a goal type such as lose, gain or maintain.
    4. Finally, enter your goal weight. If you would like, you can enter a body fat percentage goal too.

- **FITBIT.COM DASHBOARD**
    1. Begin by hovering your mouse over the bottom of the weight tile on the dashboard on fitbit.com.
    2. Then click the gear icon.
    3. Click **Goal Weight** in the weight tile.
    4. Then click **Add weight goal**.
    5. rocked by select a goal type such as lose, gain or maintain.
    6. Finally enter your goal weight. If you would like, you can enter a body fat percentage goal too. Apply the changes by clicking **Save**.

How do I change or delete my goal?

A goal may change over time. You can modify or delete goals by following these steps:

- **FITBIT APP**
    1. Start by clicking the Account icon ( ) from the dashboard of your Fitbit app.
    2. Then find **Nutrition & Body** under Goals.
    3. Finally, make changes to your goal as desired. You can delete the goal by tapping the three dots icon and tapping **Remove Weight Goal**.

- **FITBIT.COM DASHBOARD**

1. Begin by hovering your mouse over the bottom of the weight tile on the dashboard on fitbit.com.
2. Then click the gear icon.
3. Click **Goal Weight** in the weight tile.
4. Finally, make changes to your goal as desired. Click **Delete goal** and then click **Done** to delete your goal.

What should I know about food scanning?

Food scanning is a convenient way to log food. It's available with the Fitbit app for iOS, Android and Windows 10.

How do I scan a food item?

You can easily scan a food item by following these steps:

1. Start by tapping the + icon from the dashboard of your Fitbit app.
2. You must first grant access for the Fitbit app to access the required features on your mobile device if you're using Android Marshmallow.
3. Then **Scan Barcode** by tapping.
4. It's important to make sure that the item's entire barcode is within the scanning area. For items that are in the Fitbit's database, a summary will appear after a successful barcode scan.
5. You have the option to change any quantities if necessary.
6. Complete by tapping **Save**.

Why won't my item scan?

There can be many reasons for an item to be not scanning properly. The following are some common reasons why an item scan fails.

First, make sure that the item's entire barcode is within the scanning area. This is one of the most common reasons for an item not scanning.

If you continue to have trouble scanning the item, tap the 'X' to exit the scanner and then search for the food item. If the particular food item doesn't appear in the search results, you will need to create a custom food by tapping **Custom > Add Custom Food**.

Barcode scanning is currently only available for customers using the US food database. The barcode scanning option will be accessible, but it will not work if you have chosen a non-US food database. You can check which food database you're using by following these steps:

1. Start by clicking the Account icon ( ) from the dashboard of your Fitbit app.
2. Then tap **Advanced Settings**.
3. Finally, tap **Food Database** to view your food database information.

Can I add a barcode to the food database?

You can help Fitbit's food database grow by adding new food items that aren't already in the database.

When you scan an item and find out that it's not in the Fitbit's database, you will see the option to submit it as an addition.

How does Fitbit estimate how many calories I've burned?

The rate at which you burn calories while resting, in order to maintain essential body functions such as breathing, heartbeat and brain activity is called the Basal Metabolic Rate (BMR). Most interestingly, your BMR usually accounts for at least half of the calories you burn daily! You BMR will be estimated based on the physical data you enter when you set up your account such as your sex, age, height and weight.

When it comes to calorie burn estimates, Fitbit takes in consideration factors such as your BMR, the activities recorded by your tracker and any other activities you log manually.

The calorie count of your tracker resets at midnight every night. It will then begin calculating for the next day immediately.

Don't be surprised to see that you have already burned calories when you wake up in the morning! The reason behind that is your BMR. Your body still functions while you sleep and calories will be burned.

How do I track my food with Fitbit?

The food that you eat is as important as maintaining an active lifestyle. You can easily track the food that you consume with Fitbit to keep an eye on your calorie intake.

What is a food plan?

A food plan is a great way to make sure that you achieve and maintain the body weight and figure of your dreams! You can easily see how you're heading towards your goal by logging your meals each day with access to your caloric intake and burn.

You can have different goals such as lose weight, gain weight or maintain your current weight.

How do I start a food plan?

You can easily begin a food plan, log food and monitor your progress using the dashboard on fitbit.com as well as the Fitbit app. Follow these instructions to find out how to manually log an activity:

- **FITBIT APP**
    1. Start by tapping or click the Account icon ( ) from the dashboard of your Fitbit app.
    2. Then tap **Nutrition & Body** under Goals.
    3. The next step is to find the option to start a food plan under Nutrition.
    4. You can easily set up your food plan by following the onscreen instructions. Make sure that you save once you're done. If you are using the Fitbit app for iOS, you have the option to set a daily calorie goal independent of a food plan.
    5. You have the ability to change the intensity of your food plan later once you have achieved your Food goal.

- **FITBIT.COM DASHBOARD**
    1. Begin by logging into your fitbit.com dashboard.
    2. Then click **Log** found at the top and then click **Food**.
    3. You can then start by clicking the **Get Started** button in the Food Plan section.

4. Proceed by entering your starting weight, your target weight and your plan intensity when you're prompted. You will see the estimated date for reaching your goal depending on the intensity that you choose.
5. You can easily edit the intensity later by clicking the gear icon on the **Calories In vs Out** tile and clicking the pencil icon next to **Plan Intensity**. You can also change your goal weight here.

How do I monitor my progress?

Keeping an eye on your progress will help you achieve your goal on time. Your food plan helps you by providing the following information:

- An estimation of your daily calorie consumption.
- The number of calories you have burned and eaten so far in the day.
- A highly useful, real-time comparison between the calories you've consumed in your diet versus the calories you've burned through activity.
- Valuable feedback about whether you are under, within or above your plan's recommendation.
- Fitbit app for Android also provides an estimate of your daily macronutrient consumption.

It's important that you make sure that you log everything that you eat in order to achieve accurate calorie and macronutrient estimates. When you log food, the daily calorie macronutrient estimates will automatically update, showing how much you can still eat for the rest of the day while staying on track to your goal.

It's natural to vary from your daily estimate. However, make sure that it's within 50 calories of your daily estimate, to ensure that you don't drift too far away from your target. You must meet your plan's recommendation for the day when you log your last meal.

You can keep an eye on where you stand in terms of your calorie consumption using the **Calories In vs Calories Out** meter. If you app syncs regularly, the meter will continually update depending on the food logged and your activity level.

The steps that you take and activities that are logged manually will determine your activity level. When you exercise and walk through the day, your allowance of calories will adjust accordingly and let know how much more you can eat while keeping in line with your goals.

> *Putting together a food plan takes a lot of work. If you feel that you lack the nutrition knowledge to compose a good food plan, it's highly recommended that you speak with your doctor or a nutritionist before starting your new plan.*

How do I log food?

Make sure that you log anything and everything that you eat to ensure that the estimates that your tracker makes are accurate. Follow these instructions to log food with the fitbit.com dashboard:

Proceed by hovering your mouse over either the **Food Plan** or **Calories In vs. Out** tile. Then click the arrow icon in the lower right corner. You will be directed to the food log. You will be able to log your meals by entering food descriptions and quantities along with the time you consumed them.

You can also log food using the Fitbit app. Simply tap or click the + icon and tap or click **Log Food**. You are also able to log food from the home screen with the Quick Action menu using 3D Touch if your iOS mobile device supports 3D Touch.

Can I scan barcodes to log food?

This is a very convenient way to log food. The Fitbit apps support barcode scanning. Simply go to the screen where you log food and tap the barcode icon. Then hold the barcode on your food item in front of your camera.

If the type of food is recognized and belongs to your food database, you'll see "Got it". Otherwise, you will be prompted to add the food to the food database.

In the event of the food you're trying to scan isn't recognized, you will need to manually add it to your food log.

How do I delete a food entry?

It's possible that you might not eat a food that you enter into your food log. You must delete that entry if that's the case. Follow these instructions to delete a food entry:

- **FITBIT APP FOR IOS**
    1. Begin by tapping the food title from the dashboard of your Fitbit app. It's the title that says **"What have you eaten today?"** or shows you how many calories you've eaten and have left to consume today.
    2. Then find the entry that you wish to delete and slide it to the left.
    3. Finally, tap **Delete**.

- **FITBIT APP FOR ANDROID**
    1. Begin by tapping the food title from the dashboard of your Fitbit app. It's the title that says **"What have you eaten today?"** or shows you how many calories you've eaten and have left to consume today.
    2. Then tap and hold the entry you wish to delete.
    3. Finally, tap **Delete item**.

- **FITBIT APP FOR WINDOWS 10**
    1. Begin by tapping the food title from the dashboard of your Fitbit app. It's the title that says **"What have you eaten today?"** or shows you how many calories you've eaten and have left to consume today.
    2. Then tap or click the entry you wish to delete.
    3. Finally, tap or click the trashcan icon.

- **FITBIT.COM DASHBOARD**
    1. Start by going to your food log (https://www.fitbit.com/foods/log).
    2. Then hover your cursor over the entry that you wish to delete.
    3. Finally, click the "x" that appears to the left of that entry.

How do I see my macronutrients breakdown?

Understanding your macronutrient intake helps you fine tune the type of food that you consume. When you log food in the Fitbit app, you will have

access to estimate of your daily macronutrients breakdown (total carbohydrates, fat and protein consumed) as well as your caloric intake.
Your macronutrient breakdown will appear once you log food. Follow these steps to see details about your macronutrients consumption:

1. Begin by tapping the food tile (which shows your calories in vs calories remaining if you created a food plan) from the dashboard of your Fitbit app.
2. Then find your daily macronutrients breakdown as compared to your **Calories In vs Calories Out** under **Today**.
3. You can view your macronutrients breakdown over the past week by swiping the graph at the top.
4. Finally tap the expand icon in the top right to open information about your macronutrients. Then tap any particular day to see details for that day. You can close by tapping the icon again.

It's important to remember that you won't see your macronutrients breakdown if you log calories instead of food. You can find more details about the benefits of tracking macronutrients under Fitbit blog. **Note**: Fitbit blog is only available in English.

Do I have to add every ingredient in a meal?
You have the ability to create a specific meal using the dashboard on fitbit.com. This is a very convenient option, if you're cooking and want to add all the individual ingredients only once. If you cook the same meal again, you can easily add it to your food plan with one click!

1. Start by finding Favorites on the right side on the food logging page and then clicking the **Meals** tab.
2. Click the blue **"Create a meal"** link and give the meal a suitable name.
3. Then click **Save**. You can begin to add the individual foods for this meal in the Add Foods section. Every time you add each food item, click the red **Add to Meal** button.
4. Finally, click the red **I'm done** button to complete adding the meal.

You only need to do it once for a specific meal. You can add the meal again later under Custom Foods on the Fitbit app.

What Type of Food Database Does Fitbit Use?
Fitbit offers comprehensive food databases for the United States, Australia, Canada, China, France, Germany, India, Ireland, Italy, Korea, Mexico, Philippines, Singapore, Spain and the United Kingdom.

They includes simple, generic items from Fitbit's partner database, packaged items from national and regional brands as well as menu items from restaurant chains. This database is updated regularly with new foods.

Fitbit's international food database for Taiwan has simple, common items translated into the local language to make logging food easier.

How do I change the language for my food database?
To make logging food easier by having listings that suit your country, you can choose the country you want to use for your food database. Follow these steps to change the database on fitbit.com:
1. Begin by logging into your Fitbit.com dashboard. Then click the gear icon in the upper right of your screen.
2. Click **Settings** and scroll down to Preferences.
3. Then choose the food database that you prefer.
4. Finally, click **Save** to apply the changes you made.

You can change the food database on your Fitbit app. You can find this setting under Account > Advanced Settings.

What is a Calorie Deficit?
If you notice a calorie deficit, it's very good news! This simply means that you have burned more calories than you've consumed in a given day.

Aiming for calorie deficit calorie deficits is a great strategy to achieve your weight goal. You can adjust your calorie deficit target by changing the intensity of your food plan.

How do I use Fitbit to track and set goals for my water intake?

Consuming the recommended healthy amount of water every day is very important. You can use your Fitbit account to log and track your daily water consumption.

Taking it one day at a time is a good strategy. Fitbit enables you to set a water consumption goal and track your progress each day.

Logging Your Water Intake

You can easily log your water intake by following these steps:

- **FITBIT APP**
    1. Begin by tapping the water tile on the Fitbit app dashboard.
    2. Then choose an amount of water from the **Quick Add** menu.
    3. You can enter a different amount by tapping the plus icon (+) in the top right corner. Finally, enter the correct amount of water you consumed and tap **Save.**

For Fitbit users with iOS mobile devices that supports 3D Touch, it's possible to log water from the home screen with the Quick Action menu accessed by 3D Touch.

- **FITBIT.COM DASHBOARD**
    1. First, select **Log** towards the top of your screen.
    2. Then scroll to the bottom of the page and log your water intake.
    3. Finally, click **Log it**.

How do I set a goal for water intake?

Motivate yourself to drink enough water every day and track your progress by setting goals for water intake. You can achieve this by following these steps:

- **FITBIT APP**
    1. Begin by tapping or clicking the Account icon ( ) from the dashboard of your Fitbit app.
    2. Then find **Nutrition & Body** under Goals.
    3. Finally, tap **Water** and enter the number of ounces of water you plan on consuming per day. If you would like to log cups or milliliters instead, you can do so on fitbit.com.

- **FITBIT.COM DASHBOARD**
    1. Begin by hovering your mouse over the bottom of the water tile. Then, click on the gear icon.

2. Enter your desired daily water consumption goal.
3. Finally, click **Done**.

Sleep

Understanding your sleep patterns and making sure that you get enough sleep every day is an important part of healthy living. Fitbit offers a range of sleep tools to help you achieve this.

What should I know about sleep stages?

Your Fitbit recognizes that you're asleep when your body is completely at rest and unmoving. Tracking your sleep becomes more accurate if you using a Fitbit device with heart-rate tracking (except for Fitbit Charge HR and Fitbit Surge). When you are asleep, you will be cycling through various sleep stages and you will have access to these records with Fitbit.

Users of other devices can see their sleep pattern which shows the time spent awake, restless and asleep. When you move from a restful position to one that involves more movement, that state is considered as Restless. This can happen when you turn over in bed.

If you happen to be moving too much and to an extent where restful sleep isn't possible, your sleep graph will indicate that you were awake.

What are sleep stages?

Your Fitbit recognizes that you're asleep when your body is completely at rest and unmoving. Tracking your sleep becomes more accurate if you using a Fitbit device with heart-rate tracking (except for Fitbit Charge HR and Fitbit Surge). When you are asleep, you will be cycling through various sleep stages and you will have access to these records with Fitbit.

Users of other devices can see their sleep pattern which shows the time spent awake, restless and asleep. When you move from a restful position to one that involves more movement, that state is considered as Restless. This can happen when you turn over in bed.

If you happen to be moving too much and to an extent where restful sleep isn't possible, your sleep graph will indicate that you were awake.

How does my Fitbit device automatically detect my sleep stages?

If you wear your Fitbit tracker or watch to bed, they will automatically detect your sleep. When you wake up in the morning and sync your device, you'll see your sleep information on your dashboard.

If you're using Fitbit Flex 2, do not wear the pendant accessory while sleeping; classic accessory bands are the recommended for sleep tracking.

Autodetection uses your movement to define whether you're asleep or awake. If you haven't moved for about an hour, your device assumes that you're asleep.

Your Fitbit device also records additional data such as the length of time your movements which indicate of sleep behavior (such as rolling over, etc.). These records also confirm that you're asleep. Your morning movements will tell your tracker that you're awake.

In the event of you not moving for a long period of time, yet not asleep, your Fitbit device might falsely track that time as sleep. You can manually delete that time from your sleep log.

Fitbit devices with heart-rate tracking (except for Charge HR and Surge) use a combination of your movement and heart-rate patterns to estimate your sleep stages.

What does each sleep stage mean?

You will see a see a several sleep stages in your Fitbit sleep log which were named by Fitbit's sleep researchers and the National Sleep Foundation (https://sleepfoundation.org/how-sleep-works/what-happens-when-you-sleep).

Light Sleep

You can enter into a light sleep as your body unwinds and slows down. It is the entry point into sleep each night. You reach this stage within minutes of falling asleep. You tend to drift between being awake and asleep during the early part of light sleep. You can be easily awoken in this stage as you are somewhat aware of your surroundings. Your breathing and heart rate typically decrease slightly during this stage.

Your mental and physical recovery is promoted by light sleep.

Deep Sleep

You can enter into deep sleep after the first few hours of your sleep. You can wake up feeling refreshed in the morning, when you have experienced solid periods of deep sleep during the previous night. You can't be easily awoken in this stage as your body is less responsive to the outside stimuli. Your breathing becomes slowed, your muscles become more relaxed and your heart rate becomes more regular, during your deep sleep. When you get older you will notice a normal decrease in your deep sleep. However your sleeping patterns will always vary among from another person. Your physical recovery, immune system, memory and learning are promoted by deep sleep.

REM Sleep

At the initial stage of deep sleep you can enter into the first phase of REM sleep. Your REM sleep lasts for a longer period of time and it happens in the second half of the night. Your brain becomes more active at the final stage of sleep. You can dreams more during REM sleep and your eyes start to move quickly in different directions. Your breathing becomes more irregular and your heart rate increases. And you will be less active below your neck as your muscles below become inactive to avoid you from acting out in your dreams.

Your mood regulation, learning, consolidating information from the previous day to be stored in your long-term memory are being promoted during your REM sleep.

How do I see my sleep stages?
You can see the data of your sleep stages Fitbit app.

1. You can begin in the morning, by opening the Fitbit app or by clicking the sleep tile on your dashboard. You can see the details of your sleep within a few moments when your device those details to your dashboard.

2. You need to sync your dashboard to your Fitbit device's data if you see the message "Analyzing your sleep" when you tap on the sleep tile.
3. You can continue by tapping Today. And in Windows 10 by tapping Last Night.
4. You can view your stats by swiping the opened information about your sleep stages, by tapping the expand icon in the top right.
5. You can view your time spent in each stage by scrolling down to and then by tapping you can see your 30 Day Avg. You can finish by tapping Benchmark to view additional stats.

How do I use the sleep stages benchmark?

You can see get an idea about your sleep stage estimates from the previous night and also a comparison to the averages of others who are the same age range and sex using benchmark. You can read further about this on source (https://www.ncbi.nlm.nih.gov/pubmed/15586779). Benchmark is based on your published sleep data. You can see the typical range for each sleep stage shaded between the two horizontal lines, in your graph. Your sleep cycles vary naturally. And sometimes you will receive your sleep data fall outside the typical ranges. You can also compare your data from last night to your own 30 day average to analyze your sleep stages in another way. You can find your 30 day average under the 30 Day Avg tab.

How can I see the start and end times for my sleep stages?

You can gain an insight into your sleep patterns by seeing the start and end times of your different sleep stages.

- **FITBIT APP**
1. Begin by tapping or clicking the sleep tile from the Fitbit app dashboard.
2. You can see more details of your sleep stages by tapping or clicking the sleep record.
3. You can expand your sleep graph by tapping when you are using iOS or Android only.
4. You can receive information estimated sleep stages recorded at different times by tapping and holding or by tapping and clicking

the sleep graph. You can do the same by sliding your finger to see the time ranges on iOS.
- **FITBIT.COM DASHBOARD**
1. Begin by clicking the sleep tile and selecting More from the fitbit.com dashboard.
2. You can receive more details of a sleep record by clicking the particular sleep record.
3. You can get an idea about the estimated sleep stages recorded at different times by hovering your mouse over the sleep graph.

Can this tell me if I have Apnea or any other sleep disorder?

You can share your concerns about your sleep health with your doctor. You can track your sleeping patterns and notice variations with your sleep stages data. You can look into additional information about your sleep in the National Sleep Foundation (https://sleepfoundation.org/sleep-disorders-problems).

Why do I see awake minutes?

According to source (http://aasmnet.org/jcsm/Articles/030305.pdf), an adult could typically wake up briefly between 10-30 times per night. Therefore you can see awake minutes in your sleep stages. However you will not remember waking up as you are most likely fall asleep right after waking up, especially when you wake for less than 2-3 minutes at a time. Sometimes you can notice more awake minutes in your sleep stages as compared to other nights. in such nights you will notice that your sleep was restless.

You can log the times that you have spent awake, restless, and asleep, in your Fitbit and track those data. Aside from these entries, your Fitbit also uses heart rate and other data, so you can track your sleep in order to estimate your sleep stages. With the combination of all these data you can have a better sense of your sleep cycles.

With this change, you can notice more awake minutes in sleep your stages than in your previous sleep data. You can edit your, you can edit your sleep goal to make sure that you still meet your Fitbit goals.

Your sleep stages aren't affected by the sleep sensitivity setting on your device.

Why don't I see sleep stages today?

You can see your sleep pattern with the times that you have been asleep, restless, and awake, instead of sleep stages. This can happen due to a few scenarios:

- You could've slept in a position that prevents your device from getting a consistent heart-rate reading or you could've worn it too loosely. To avoid this you can wear your device higher on your wrist, about 2-3 finger widths above your wrist bone and your Fitbit band should feel secure but not too tight.
- Instead of simply wearing your device to bed, you could've used the Begin Sleep Now option in the Fitbit app.
- When you had a sleep that is less than 3 hours.
- When your device's battery is critically low.

You can receive more information on reasons for why you are seeing your sleep pattern by tapping or clicking the sleep record.

Why don't I see sleep stages for naps?

You can't include your nap data to estimate your sleep stages because your device needs at least 3 hours of sleep data to estimate your sleep stages.

Can I edit my sleep stages data?

You can manually edit your sleep log when the start and end times of your sleep are incorrect, to get a better reflection of your time asleep. You will notice gaps at the start or end times of your sleep stages when you extend your time asleep.

What are some tips for getting a good night's sleep?

You can take several steps to enhance your chances for getting a good night's sleep. You can stick to a sleep schedule, avoid naps in the afternoon, practice a relaxing bedtime routine, and exercise daily to help you in getting a good night's sleep. You can find other recommendations in the National Sleep Foundation (https://sleepfoundation.org/sleep-tools-tips/healthy-sleep-tips).

You can also use several Fitbit tools to achieve this. In the Fitbit app you can set a sleep schedule to maintain a more consistent pattern of sleep.

You can also use the sleep insights and set a bedtime reminder in the Fitbit app, not only to get a good night' sleep but also to learn about your sleep habits.

How do I change my sleep history?

Can I manually log sleep?
Your Fitbit device can automatically start and stop your sleep log. You can use the app to start and stop sleep tracking when sleep detection is inaccurate. However this can't be applied if you use a Fitbit device with heart-rate tracking to detect your sleep stages.

1. Begin by tapping the sleep tile from the Fitbit app dashboard. You can recognize this tile as it says "How did you sleep?" or it is the tile that shows your sleeping time in hours and minutes.
2. You can track your sleep by tapping the + icon and then by tapping the Begin Sleep Now. Then you can minimize the app and go to sleep.
3. You can finish by tapping I'm Awake and selecting View Summary to see a summary of your sleep once you wake up.

The method to edit your sleep logs in your Fitbit app for Windows 10. You won't be able to do this manually.

Why does my sleep graph say I was asleep when I wasn't?
Your Fitbit can auto detect sleep when the device is off your wrist. But occasionally these tend to record a sleep log when you are awake. You can delete such sleep logs on your dashboard.

Why does my sleep graph say I was awake when I wasn't?
You tend to toss and turn during your sleep. Your sleep is not considered total rest with these unconscious movements. You can set your sleep tracking mode to sensitive by going to the Sleep Sensitivity setting, when your reported number of awake minutes is excessively high. You can have a general overview of your sleep patterns using a normal setting. But you won't find this setting when you use a Fitbit device with heart-rate tracking to detect your sleep stages.

How do I edit a sleep log?
You can get a better reflection of your sleeping patterns by editing the sleep log. Your Fitbit device with heart-rate tracking (except Charge HR)

will give gaps at the start or end times of your sleeping stages, when you extend your sleeping time.

Edit your sleep log by choosing your mobile device.

- **FITBIT APP FOR IOS AND WINDOWS 10**
1. Begin by tapping the sleep tile From the Fitbit app dashboard. You can recognize this tile as it says "How did you sleep?" or it is the tile that shows your sleeping time in hours and minutes.
2. You can edit your sleep log by selecting the sleep log you want to edit.
3. Then you can continue editing by tapping the three dots and selection the option to edit.
4. Finish by adjusting the time you went to sleep or the time you woke up and saving your changes.
- **FITBIT APP FOR ANDROID**
1. Begin by tapping the sleep tile From the Fitbit app dashboard. You can recognize this tile as it says "How did you sleep?" or it is the tile that shows your sleeping time in hours and minutes.
2. You can edit your sleep log by selecting the sleep log you want to edit.
3. Finish by tapping the pencil icon in the top right corner and adjusting the time you went to sleep or the time you woke up and then by saving your changes.

How do I delete a sleep log?

You can delete any sleep log that you don't need n your sleep history.

Delete your sleep log by choosing your mobile device.

- **FITBIT APP FOR IOS AND ANDROID**
1. Begin by tapping the sleep tile From the Fitbit app dashboard. You can recognize this tile as it says "How did you sleep?" or it is the tile that shows your sleeping time in hours and minutes.
2. Delete your sleep log by swipe left on the log you want to erase and tapping Delete.
- **FITBIT APP FOR WINDOWS 10**
1. Begin by tapping the sleep tile From the Fitbit app dashboard. You can recognize this tile as it says "How did you sleep?" or it is the tile that shows your sleeping time in hours and minutes.

2. You can select the sleep log that you want to delete by tapping it.
3. Finish by tapping the three dots and then by tapping delete.

What should I know about setting a sleep schedule?

You can maintain a more consistent pattern of sleep and meet your sleep goal by setting a sleep schedule in your Fitbit app.

Why should I maintain a consistent sleep schedule?

According to source (https://www.nlm.nih.gov/medlineplus/magazine/issues/summer12/articles/summer12pg20.html), you can sleep better and get more sleep when you wake up and go to bed at a consistent time. Your long-term health can be compromised with an insufficient sleep. As source (http://www.nhlbi.nih.gov/health/health-topics/topics/sdd/why) states, you are more likely to have increased rates of chronic diseases and conditions, when you consistently fail to get enough sleep. You can set a sleep schedule to help you achieve a healthy sleep cycle.

How does Fitbit estimate how much sleep I need?

Data of source (https://sleepfoundation.org/media-center/press-release/national-sleep-foundation-recommends-new-sleep-times) suggests that an adult needs to get seven to nine hours of sleep per night. However, you can set your sleep goal attainable and to meet your individual needs.

Your Fitbit estimate your sleep goal by averaging your five or more sleep logs. When you don't get enough sleep or when you want to set a different goal, you can manually adjust your goal.

You can start by begin by estimating your sleeping hours on a typical night, when you haven't tracked your sleep before. Your Fitbit set your goal based on that estimate, when your estimation can be considered as enough sleep. You can always manually adjust the goal when the estimation doesn't provide enough sleep or when you want to set a different goal.

Do I have to set a bedtime and wake-up time target?

You can achieve a more consistent sleep cycle when you set the both bedtime and wake-up time. But you can also set either bedtime or wake-up time too.

How are my bedtime and wake-up time targets calculated?
Your Fitbit can estimate your wake-up time target, based on your typical wake up time, when you have five or more sleep logs. Then you can set your bedtime as a default in your Fitbit, in order to meet your sleep goal. However, you can manually change one or both of these times. You can manually set targets for both the bedtime and wake-up times when you have fewer than five sleep logs.

How do I meet my bedtime and wake-up time targets?
You can sleep or wake up within 30 minutes of your target in order to meet your target. You receive a star in the sleep schedule graph when you meet your target. You won't receive a when you only meet one target after setting the both bedtime and wake-up time targets.

How do I set or change my bedtime or wake-up time target?
You can set, change, or remove a bedtime or a wake-up time target:

- **FITBIT APP FOR IOS AND ANDROID**
    1. Begin by tapping the sleep tile from the Fitbit app dashboard. You can recognize this tile as it says "How did you sleep?" or it is the tile that shows how many hours and minutes that you slept when you have tracked sleep the night before.
    2. You can continue by tapping the gear icon in the top right.
    3. Then you can set or edit targets. You can remove a target by tapping the three dots in the top right of your screen.
    4. Finally tap Done.
- **FITBIT APP FOR WINDOWS 10**
1. Begin by tapping or clicking the sleep tile from the Fitbit app dashboard. It's the title that says "How did you sleep?" or shows how many hours and minutes you slept if you tracked sleep the night before.
2. Then tap or click the moon icon on the bottom.
3. You can now set or edit your targets. You can remove a target by tapping the three dots in the bottom right.
4. Finally, tap Save.

Do I need to set a bedtime target to receive a bedtime reminder?
Containing a consistent sleep schedule is a great way to make sure that you're on track for a healthy life. You can set a bedtime reminder to help you maintain a consistent sleep schedule. The bedtime reminders let you know when it's time to call it a day. You can have a bedtime reminder even without setting a bedtime target.

Health

What is female health tracking in the Fitbit app?

Why should I use the female health tracking feature in the Fitbit app?
You need to use the female health tracking feature in your Fitbit app because tracking your cycle can empower you to thoroughly understand what happens in your body, your recurring irregularities and your menstrual patterns, which are linked to everyday activities like sleep and exercise.

What is a menstrual cycle?
Your menstrual cycle is a recurring cycle. This happens when the lining of your uterus thickens as a preparation for a possible pregnancy and then it sheds if you are not pregnant. For more information, see, source (https://www.womenshealth.gov/glossary#m). You get your monthly bleeding occurs with the shedding of the uterine lining. This is what you know as getting your period. The source (https://www.mayoclinic.org/healthy-lifestyle/womens-health/in-depth/menstrual-cycle/art-20047186) has further details in this topic. According to source (https://www.ncbi.nlm.nih.gov/pubmed/22350580), a typical menstrual cycles lasts from 21 to 35 days, with an average of a 28-day cycle and typically periods last 2-8 days, with an average of 5 days. Your menstrual cycle is counted from the first day of your period to the day before your next period, as stated in source (https://www.womenshealth.gov/menstrual-cycle/your-menstrual-cycle).

What is a fertile window and ovulation?

As mentioned in source (https://www.mayoclinic.org/healthy-lifestyle/getting-pregnant/in-depth/female-fertility/art-20045887), fertility refers to your ability to conceive a biological child. Your fertile window is the portion of your menstrual cycle when you're most fertile, you can find out more details on this from, source (https://www.ncbi.nlm.nih.gov/pubmed/7477165). Fertile windows typically span 6 days with ovulation occurring on the 6th day. But your fertile windows can be longer or shorter than this. Ovulation occurs when one of your ovaries releases an egg into a fallopian tube. In your Fitbit app, the fertile window spans 7 days to interpret your variations in the time of day that ovulation occurs. You can read more about this in source (https://www.bmj.com/content/321/7271/1259.short).

What are predictions in the female health tracking feature?
You can see the predictions of future periods and fertile windows, based on the information you provide about your menstrual cycle.

How does the Fitbit app predict my periods and fertile windows?
You receive your predictions of your period, fertile window and ovulation. This happens as a result of using your period and cycle length information, in an algorithm, which is being used by your Fitbit. Your Fitbit uses the typical 28-day cycle and 5-day period, as the starting point for estimations, when you don't provide all the required information about your cycle. You can always notice your fertile window as 7 days in the Fitbit app. You can personalize your period and fertile window predictions as you log your period consistently.

You can edit the average cycle length and period length that you provided during setup. However, these settings will only affect your initial predictions.

How accurate are predictions?
Initially, your predictions are made by considering the average cycle and period lengths you provide during setup. Your predictions become more accurate with time as you log your period consistently.

What are trends in the female health tracking feature?
You can view your cycle trends to see patterns in your cycle length, period length, ovulation, and fertile windows.

Can female health tracking tell me if I have an unusual cycle or any other disorder?
You can always track your patterns and notice variations using the female health tracking.

You may get irregular periods due to a several factors. Some of the common causes include your usage of hormonal birth control, pregnancy, and excessive physical activity. Find out more information in source (https://my.clevelandclinic.org/health/diseases/14633-abnormal-menstruation-periods). The source (https://www.mayoclinic.org/healthy-lifestyle/womens-health/in-depth/menstrual-cycle/art-20047186?pg=2) goes on to state that a "normal" period is whatever is normal for you and your cycle.

You can consult your doctor when you have any concerns about your cycle.

When you use certain types of contraception, like; extended-cycle birth control pills and intrauterine devices (IUDs), those will alter your menstrual cycle. You can read further about this in this source (https://www.mayoclinic.org/healthy-lifestyle/womens-health/in-depth/menstrual-cycle/art-20047186). You need to talk to your health care provider about what to expect before using such contraception methods.

You can use the female health tracking feature to track your cycle and details and to recognize patterns even when you are using birth control or otherwise have an altered cycle. In such an instance you turn off predictions in the female health settings and manually log your periods into your Fitbit device.

Why do I need to add my birth control method?
As your birth control method can affect your cycle, it is better if you add your birth control method to log the details.

Can I share my period data?
To achieve more personalized care you can share your female health data with your doctor. This will help your doctor to get a clearer picture of your menstrual cycle. But at this time, you won't be able to directly share your

female health tracking data from your Fitbit app with anyone, including your partner.

Your Fitbit is designed in a way to protect your privacy and to keep your data safe. There is a combination of technical, administrative and physical controls to maintain the security of your data.

Can I use my female health data for family planning?
Your female health tracking helps you to learn more about your cycle and recognize its' trends. Even though your Fitbit provides you information about your estimated fertile window, you need to always talk to your doctor when it comes to conceiving and pregnancy.

Can my partner use the female health tracking feature to participate in family planning?

You can't share your female health data directly from the Fitbit app. But you can review your data with your partner or your health care professional when you track your menstrual cycle information and details in the Fitbit app.

Your female health tracking is getting switched off by default if you are male Fitbit app user.

Can I log ovulation test results in the Fitbit app?
You can only log your periods and cycle details in order to see your estimated fertile windows and ovulation days. You can't log your ovulation tests as those are not supported at this time.

Can I log pregnancy test results in the Fitbit app?
You can't log pregnancy test results at this time. You can continue using female health tracking during your pregnancy, by turning off the predictions.

You can keep logging details, like; headaches or bleeding and track your female health information. You need to talk to your doctor whenever you have any concerns.

Is female health tracking available on a child account in a Fitbit family account?
You can't have female health tracking in your Fitbit app for children on family accounts, at this time.

How do I use the Fitbit app to track my period?

What information can I track in the Fitbit female health feature?

You can follow your cycle, log periods, record details, and analyze the trends in your cycle at a glance with the female health tracking in your Fitbit app.

How do I set up the female health tracking feature in the Fitbit app?

1. Begin by adding the female health tile to your Fitbit app dashboard if you don't already have it.
2. You can continue by clicking the female health tracking tile from the Fitbit app dashboard.
3. By following the on-screen instructions you can set up your female health tracking. You need to answer the series of questions that you are being asked about your menstrual cycle. This initial information of yours is used to make predictions about your future period and fertile windows. You can always edit or update your information later.

- You can find the approximate date your last period started on the calendar of your app.
- You can edit your average period and cycle lengths, by tapping the + or – icons, in order to add or subtract days.
- You can turn on notifications and receive reminders on your phone about the predictions of when you will start your period.

How do I add or remove the female health tracking tile in the Fitbit app?
Making the female health tile visible:

1. Begin by tapping Edit at the bottom of the dashboard, from your Fitbit app dashboard.

2. By tapping the + icon in the top left corner of the female health tile, you can make female health tile visible.
3. Finish by clicking Done.

Making the female health tile invisible:

1. Begin by tapping Edit at the bottom of the dashboard, from your Fitbit app dashboard.
2. By tapping the x or - icon in the top left corner of the female health tile, you can make female health tile invisible.
3. Finish by clicking Done.

How do I add, edit or delete a period in the Fitbit app?

Adding or editing a period:

1. Begin by tapping the female health tile from your Fitbit app dashboard.
2. Then you can tap or click the start date of a period on the calendar.
3. By clicking the pencil icon (✏), you can add or edit you period (you can also tap and hold a date on the calendar). You can see the entire period on the calendar based on your average period length when you turn on the predictions.
4. You can adjust your period length on the calendar, by tapping the first or last day of a period and then sliding your finger across the dates.
5. Finish by tapping Save.

Deleting a period:

1. Begin by tapping the female health tile from your Fitbit app dashboard.
2. You can continue by tapping or clicking a date on the calendar inside the period that you wish to delete.
3. You can finish by tapping the pencil icon (✏) and selecting Delete.

How do I confirm a predicted period in the Fitbit app?

You will be asked to confirm whether your period has started, during your predicted period. You can select Yes to confirm that your period has started or Not Yet to confirm that your period hasn't started. You can adjust the dates before you confirm your period by tap Edit.

When you confirm your predicted period, it becomes your confirmed period. Your period prediction remains on your calendar when you don't confirm your predicted period. After the last day of the prediction window passes, the entire predicted period shifts to the next day. Your calendar doesn't update until after midnight.

How do I log or delete female health details?

1. Begin by tapping or clicking the female health tile from the Fitbit app dashboard.
2. You can then tap or click a date on the calendar.
3. You can continue by tapping the plus icon (⊕)
4. Finally you can tap or click details to log those. And you can delete a detail, by tapping it and by making check mark disappear.
5. Finish by tapping Save.

Can I edit a fertile window in the Fitbit app?

You can't still edit fertile windows in your Fitbit. According to the menstrual cycle data you enter your estimated fertile window automatically adjusts.

How do I read the female health tracking calendar in the Fitbit app?

You can view the calendar with your cycle information by tapping or clicking the female health tile from the Fitbit app dashboard. You can identify various stages of your cycle with the different colors on the calendar.

You can review the female health details you logged for that day and other information by tapping or clicking on a date.

Please note that the gray shading indicates a month, not your cycle.

Information about the calendar icons and colors:

Icon	Description	Meaning
●	Confirmed period	Solid pink indicates a confirmed period. If you don't have your period, you can edit

Icon	Description	Meaning
		the dates.
	Predicted period	Light pink indicates a predicted period.
	Estimated fertile window	Solid blue indicates an estimated fertile window.
	Estimated ovulation day	A flower inside a fertile window indicates your estimated ovulation day.
	Confirmed period & estimated fertile window	Solid pink and blue overlapping to form purple means your predicted period and estimated fertile window overlap.
	Selected day ring	A circle indicates the selected date.
	Today ring	The Today ring indicates the current date.
	Logged detail dot	A dot underneath a date on the calendar indicates you logged female health details for that day.

How do I change the day of the week my calendar starts to Monday?

1. Begin by tapping the account icon ( ) from the Fitbit app dashboard.
2. You can scroll down and tap on Advanced Settings to continue.
3. Your female health calendar updates automatically when you tap or click Start Week On and choose which day you want your weeks to begin.

What should I know before tracking my period with Fitbit?
TIPS

- You can add or edit a period by tapping and holding your finger on a date on the calendar, instead of tapping the pencil icon.
- You can always log your period consistently for receive more personalized predictions.

Why can't I log or edit a period or female health details in the Fitbit app?

You will receive an error when your period doesn't meet certain requirements and you won't be able to log your period.

- You can only add or edit current or past periods and details.
- Your period need to last at least 1 day.
- Also your period must be less than 11 days. You can consider logging flow intensity details when your period is longer.
- Your cycle must be at least 11 days, and there must be a gap of at least 1 day between your logged periods. When you experience a gap in bleeding during your period, it's still considered 1 period.

You can't log a period in the future or a period with less than a one-day gap between periods. In such instances the pencil icon (✏) will be unavailable in your device. Your period logging or editing entries need to meet all of the requirements for you to see the pencil icon on your device.

How can I see trends in my period data?
You can review your average period and cycle lengths, average estimated ovulation day, and graphs of your past cycles by tapping the female health tile and then by tapping the Trends at the top from the Fitbit app dashboard.

How can I edit my female health settings?
You can update information about your cycle, including your period length, your cycle length and your birth control method. Not only that you can choose whether to show your period predictions and receive notifications.

1. Begin by tapping or clicking the female health tile from the Fitbit app dashboard.
2. You can adjust your female health settings as needed by clicking the gear icon (⚙).

Can the Fitbit app remind me when my period will start?

You can turn on period notifications in order to receive reminders about your upcoming predicted periods. In that way you can receive a notification on your phone 2 days before your period starts and on the first day of your predicted period. You will also be able to receive a reminder on your Fitbit watch in Fitbit Today. You can't receive any notification when you haven't turn on the period notifications.

Can I edit my average cycle or period length?

You can always edit the average cycle length and period length that you provided during setup. However, these changes in settings only affect your initial predictions.

You need to remind a several factors:

- You can change your average period length and adjust it to the length of your initial period predictions. For an example, you will see a change in your predictions when you change your average period length from 5 days to 8 days.
- You can also edit your average cycle length and adjust it to the length of your entire cycle. The predictions for your fertile window and ovulation day adjust based on the length of your cycle.

Changing your setup values for average cycle or period length:

1. Begin by tapping or clicking the female health tile from the Fitbit app dashboard.
2. You can continue by tapping the gear icon (⚙).
3. You can adjust the number by tapping Period Length or Cycle Length.
4. Finish by confirming your changes.

What do the female health icons mean on the Fitbit app dashboard?

In your Fitbit app the female health tile icon changes depending on where

Image	Meaning
	If you haven't logged any periods or you aren't using predictions, you see the female health tile with no cycle information.
Female Health Tracking and Trends	
	Read the cycle ring (the outer circle) clockwise. It represents your cycle. The pink section represents your period, and the blue section represents your estimated fertile window. The dot, which can be black or white, shows where you are in your cycle.
2 days until next period	The black dot on the cycle ring shows where you are in your cycle and that you are approaching your predicted period. The empty period icon in the center ( ) indicates you don't currently have your period.
1 day until period ends	The white dot on the cycle ring shows where you are within your predicted or confirmed period window. The filled period icon in the center ( ) indicates that today is a predicted or confirmed period day.
4 days until fertile window	The black dot on the cycle ring and the empty fertile window icon in the center ( ) indicate you had your period and are approaching your estimated fertile window.
3 days left in fertile window	The white dot on the cycle ring and the filled fertile window icon in the center ( ) indicate you're in your estimated fertile window.
1 day of period left & 4 days fertile	The white dot inside the purple overlap on the cycle ring and the overlapped period and fertile window icons ( ) indicate you are in your predicted period and estimated fertile windows at the same time.

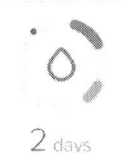

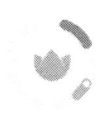

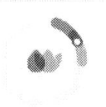

Why do my period and fertile windows overlap?
You can notice purple shading on the calendar when your estimated fertile window and period overlap on the same day.

How do I log bleeding between my periods?
You might experience a bleeding before your period, this is known as breakthrough bleeding or spotting. In such a case you can track it by logging flow intensity details.

Do I see a period on the Fitbit female health calendar if I log flow details?
Your calendar unfortunately doesn't add a period when you log your flow intensity details.

How do I confirm my period if it arrives early?
You can add your period as a new period if it arrives early. Your future predictions automatically adjust accordingly.

How can I see my period information on my Fitbit watch?
You can see the period information from swiping up from the clock face and by scrolling until you see your female health information.

You can only see your female health data on your watch, when you have set up female health tracking in your Fitbit app and log at least 1 period. You can delete all your female health data in your Fitbit app when you don't want to see period information on your Fitbit watch. By syncing your watch to you will be able to see the most recent information.

Can I see my cycle information on the Fitbit.com dashboard?
Unfortunately, you can only receive female health tracking in the Fitbit app for iOS, Android and Windows 10 at this time.

How do I add previously tracked cycle information to the Fitbit app?
You can manually add data from cycles you tracked outside the Fitbit app. But at this time, you can't import data from other apps.

Fitbit Pay
You can find Fitbit Pay which was originally launched on the Fitbit Ionic and now on the Versa. You can make mobile payments from your wrist via

Fitbit Pay. With this, you can you can hop into a corner store to buy water, while you're out for a run, without needing your wallet or phone.

Everything you need to know about Fitbit Pay.

What is Fitbit Pay?

You have heard about Apple Pay or Google Pay. Now it's time to know about Fitbit Pay. Fitbit Pay is basically the same thing as Apple Pay or Google Pay. You can find it on the Fitbit Ionic and now it's also available on the new Fitbit Versa.

You can make payments on the go, right from your wrist using the buil – in NFC chip in your Fitbit. It is a mobile payment system that works with all contactless payment readers. Therefore like mentioned before, you can pay for your water, mid run.

According to Fitbit said (https://investor.fitbit.com/press/press-releases/press-release-details/2017/Fitbit-Launches-Ionic-the-Ultimate-Health-and-Fitness-Smartwatch/default.aspx) it's Ionic's NFC chip lets you to effortlessly pay for items right from your device and leave your wallet and phone at home when you go for a run. And also this NFC chip will one day make it possible to have a keyless and card-less access to buildings, hotels, sporting venues, and transportation via using your Fitbit in the future.

What banks support Fitbit Pay?

Fitbit pay supports a number of banks located all over the word. That means you'll be able to use Fitbit Pay cards to make mobile payments using your watch.

You can find the full list of compatible banks for the US here:

- American Express
- Bank of America
- Boeing Employees Credit Union - Debit
- Capital One - Credit
- CedarStone Bank
- Citizens Equity First Credit Union (Mastercard)
- Commerce Bank
- Fisher National Bank (Mastercard)

- First National Bank of Spearman (Mastercard)
- First Tech Federal Credit Union (Mastercard)
- Peoples National Bank of Kewanee (Mastercard)
- Security Service Federal Credit Union
- Sun Community Federal Credit Union (Mastercard)
- The Colorado Bank & Trust Company of La Junta (Mastercard)
- Triad Bank (Mastercard)
- U.S. Bank
- Wells Fargo
- VACU (Mastercard)

You can find the full list of compatible banks for the UK here:

- boon by Wirecard
- Santander (Mastercard)
- Danske Bank (Mastercard)
- Starling Bank (Mastercard)

You can find the list of supported countries here:

- Australia
- Canada
- Denmark
- Finland
- Ireland
- Italy
- New Zealand
- Norway
- Singapore
- Spain
- Sweden
- Switzerland
- United Kingdom
- United State of America

Furthermore, you can find the full list of the supported banks on Fitbit's site right here (https://www.fitbit.com/fitbit-pay/banks).

How does Fitbit Pay work?

You can add your card, then go to a store and make the payment by long pressing the left-hand button and holding your Ionic watch next to contactless reader at checkout. It's that simple.

Adding your credit or debit card

You can to add any credit card or debit card from any eligible "top issuing banks in over 10 markets across the globe", like; your US American Express card or your Mastercard and Visa credit and debit cards.

For you to be using the cards from American Express, Mastercard, and Visa you will require your bank support. You can't connect your card without your bank's support. Both Apple Pay and Android Pay have taken quite a while to get banks onboard with their respective mobile payment technologies, so it may take a while for your bank to be supported for your Fitbit.

You can add the details in the Fitbit app on your phone when your bank is supported. You will notice a verification in details before being synced to your Ionic or Versa watch. You can complete the process when the watch is connected via Bluetooth. It is simple, and it won't take a long to complete.

Go to a store

You can use Fitbit Pay at anywhere that accepts contactless payments, which includes over a million stores. You can look for the contactless payments symbol (https://en.wikipedia.org/wiki/Contactless_payment) near card readers during checkout.

Now, although you won't find announcements in stores saying that they will accept Fitbit Pay payments, the following US and UK stores accept contactless payments and work with Apple Pay as well as Android Pay:

- Starbucks, Babies-R-Us, Bloomingdales, Disney, Duane Reade, Macy's, McDonalds, Nike, Petco, Staples, Subway, Toys-R-Us, Unleashed, Walgreens, Whole Foods, Boots, Bill's, Dune, Waitrose, M&S, Wagamama, Nando's, Liberty, and Lidl

If you are in a Fitbit user in UK, you can simply use the Fitbit Pay by tapping your contactless card on the reader. You can activate payment on the watch and then pay by placing your watch next to the reader when you see the symbol.

You can see a tick on the watch display when the payment goes through. And also you will receive a notification from your Fitbit app to tell you what you've paid for. You don't have risk of skimming from your watch without you knowing because you have to deliberately activate the payment on the watch for each payment.

Which Fitbit devices work with Fitbit Pay?
You can use Fitbit Pay with Fitbit Ionic and the Fitbit Versa.

Anything else you should know?
You will only need any other authentication, such as a fingerprint scan, only for large payments. In the UK, you can make contactless payment transactions up to £30, while some banks in the US limit it to $50.

Printed in Great Britain
by Amazon